DIY NATURAL SKINCARE

Creating Homemade Skincare Products Using Natural Ingredients

ELARA FINCH

Contents

Introduction 1

Importance of natural skincare 1

Benefits of DIY skincare 2

Overview of the book's purpose and structure 3

Acknowledgment 4

Chapter 1: Understanding Natural Skincare 6

Definition and principles of natural skincare 6

Benefits of using natural ingredients 8

Common harmful ingredients to avoid 9

Chapter 2: Getting Started with DIY Skincare 12

Essential tools and equipment 12

Importance of proper hygiene and safety measures 14

Tips for sourcing high-quality natural ingredients 16

Chapter 3: Key Ingredients for DIY Skincare 18

Overview of beneficial natural ingredients 18

Properties and benefits of each ingredient 19

Where to find and how to store them 21

Chapter 4: Basic DIY Skincare Recipes 23

CLEANSERS AND TONERS 23

Honey Cleansing Face Wash 25

Oatmeal Cleansing Milk 27

Green Tea Facial Cleanser 29

Yogurt and Cucumber Cleanser 31

Coconut Oil Cleanser 33

Honey and Lemon Cleanser 35

Cucumber and Mint Cleanser..................................37

Yogurt and Turmeric Cleanser 39

Coconut Milk and Aloe Vera Cleanser....................41

Papaya Cleanser...43

Apple Cider Vinegar Toner 45

Cucumber and Witch Hazel Toner 47

Rosewater and Aloe Vera Toner 49

Green Tea Toner..51

Chamomile Toner...53

Lavender Toner 55

Mint Toner...57

MOISTURIZERS AND SERUMS 59

Coconut Oil Moisturizer...61

Shea Butter Moisturizer...63

Aloe Vera Gel Moisturizer 65

Honey Moisturizer..67

Olive Oil Moisturizer 69

Cocoa Butter Moisturizer 71

Avocado Moisturizer..73

Jojoba Oil Moisturizer..75

Rosehip Oil Moisturizer 77

Cucumber Moisturizer 79

Vitamin C Serum 81

Rosehip Oil Serum 83

Frankincense and Jojoba Serum 85

Argan Oil Serum 87

Grapeseed Oil Serum 89

FACE MASKS AND SCRUBS................................. 91

Honey and Yogurt Face Mask................................. 93

Oatmeal and Banana Face Mask 95

Avocado and Honey Face Mask 97

Turmeric and Yogurt Face Mask 99

Cucumber and Aloe Vera Face Mask 101

Sugar and Olive Oil Scrub 103

Coffee Grounds and Coconut Oil Scrub 105

Sea Salt and Grapefruit Scrub 107

Brown Sugar and Honey Scrub............................. 109

Almond Meal and Yogurt Scrub 111

LIP BALMS AND BODY BUTTERS 113

Coconut Oil and Beeswax Lip Balm..................... 115

Shea Butter and Almond Oil Lip Balm.................. 116

Honey and Olive Oil Lip Balm 117

Cocoa Butter and Vitamin E Lip Balm 118

Shea Butter and Coconut Oil Body Butter............. 119

Cocoa Butter and Jojoba Oil Body Butter.............. 121

Mango Butter and Sweet Almond Oil Body Butter 123

Avocado Butter and Argan Oil Body Butter 125

Hair care products...127

Coconut Oil Hair Mask 129

Apple Cider Vinegar Rinse 131

Avocado and Banana Hair Mask.........................132

Aloe Vera Gel Hair Gel.....................................133

Olive Oil and Honey Deep Conditioning Treatment 135

Chapter 5: Advanced DIY Skincare Recipes 137

ANTI-AGING TREATMENTS................................137

Hyaluronic Acid Serum 140

Glycolic Acid Peel...142

Retinol Face Serum 144

Collagen-Boosting Mask.....................................146

Hydrating Facial Oil...148

ACNE-FIGHTING SOLUTIONS 150

Salicylic Acid Peel 152

Bentonite Clay Mask 154

Garlic and Yogurt Spot Treatment 156

Neem Oil and Aloe Vera Gel Spot Treatment.......158

Tea Tree Oil Spot Treatment 160

Natural remedies for specific skin conditions 162

Tea Tree Oil Spot Treatment for acne-prone skin: 164

Honey and Avocado Moisturizing Face Mask for dry and dull skin: 164

Chamomile and Oatmeal Soothing Face Mask for irritated or sensitive skin: 164

Lemon Juice and Honey Brightening Treatment for hyperpigmentation: 164

Bentonite or Kaolin Clay Mask for oily skin: 164

Cucumber and Mint Cooling Toner for cooling and refreshing the skin: 165

Aloe Vera and Coconut Oil After-Sun Soothing Gel for sunburned skin: 165

Green Tea and Rice Water Facial Cleanser for brightening and cleansing: 165

Turmeric and Yogurt Face Scrub for exfoliating and brightening: 165

Rosewater and Witch Hazel Toning Mist for balancing and toning: 166

Sunscreen and natural SPF options 167

Zinc Oxide Sunscreen: 167

Red Raspberry Seed Oil: 167

Carrot Seed Oil: 168

DIY Sunscreen Bars: 168

Additional Sun Protection Measures: 168

Chapter 6: Customizing and Adapting Recipes 169

Understanding skin types and specific needs 169

Modifying recipes for different skin concerns 172

Creating personalized skincare routines 174

Chapter 7: Troubleshooting and Common FAQs 178

Addressing common issues in DIY skincare 178

Troubleshooting ingredient interactions 182

Answering frequently asked questions 185

Chapter 8: Sustainability and Eco-Friendly Practices 189

Importance of sustainable skincare choices 189

Tips for reducing waste and packaging 193

Exploring eco-friendly alternatives 196

Chapter 9: Safety Considerations and Allergies 199

Identifying potential allergies and sensitivities 199

Patch testing and safety precautions 204

Consulting professionals when needed 207

Chapter 10: Incorporating Skincare into a Healthy Lifestyle 210

Importance of a holistic approach to skincare 210

Balancing skincare with nutrition and exercise 213

Self-care practices for overall well-being 216

Conclusion 218

Recap of key points and takeaways 218

Encouragement to start the journey of DIY natural skincare 220

Final thoughts and resources for further exploration. 223

About the Author 225

INTRODUCTION

Importance of natural skincare

The importance of natural skincare lies in its ability to provide safe and effective alternatives to conventional products. By opting for natural ingredients, we minimize exposure to potentially harmful chemicals, reducing the risk of skin irritation and long-term health effects. Natural skincare promotes healthier skin by nourishing and rejuvenating it with vitamins, minerals and antioxidants. Additionally, embracing natural skincare supports sustainable practices, such as eco-friendly packaging and ethical sourcing. By choosing natural skincare, we prioritize our well-being, contribute to environmental preservation, and make conscious choices that align with our values of safety, health and sustainability.

Benefits of DIY skincare

DIY skincare offers a multitude of benefits that make it increasingly popular among individuals seeking a personalized and natural approach to skincare. First and foremost, DIY skincare allows complete control over the ingredients used, ensuring the exclusion of harmful chemicals commonly found in commercial products. This promotes healthier skin and reduces the risk of adverse reactions. Additionally, DIY skincare is cost-effective, as homemade products often use affordable ingredients that can be easily sourced. The flexibility to customize recipes to individual skin types and concerns is another advantage, allowing for tailored solutions. DIY skincare also fosters creativity and empowerment, as individuals can experiment with various ingredients and formulations. Furthermore, making skincare products at home promotes sustainability by reducing packaging waste and environmental impact. Ultimately, DIY skincare offers a holistic and empowering experience that nurtures skin health while aligning with personal values of naturalness, cost-effectiveness and eco-consciousness.

Overview of the book's purpose and structure

"DIY Natural Skincare: Creating Homemade Skincare Products Using Natural Ingredients" provides a comprehensive guide to crafting your own skincare products. It offers step-by-step instructions, essential ingredient knowledge and customizable recipes. With a focus on natural ingredients, the book promotes healthier skincare choices while emphasizing the importance of sustainability and eco-friendly practices. The structure includes chapters on understanding natural skincare, getting started with DIY skincare, key ingredients, basic and advanced recipes, troubleshooting and incorporating skincare into a holistic lifestyle.

This book aims to empower readers to take control of their skincare routine, embrace natural ingredients and achieve healthier, radiant skin.

ACKNOWLEDGMENT

I would like to express my deepest gratitude and appreciation to all those who have contributed to the creation of this book, "DIY Natural Skincare: Creating Homemade Skincare Products Using Natural Ingredients."

First and foremost, I would like to thank the readers and skincare enthusiasts who have shown immense interest and support for this book. Your enthusiasm for natural skincare and your desire to explore the world of DIY skincare have inspired me to compile this comprehensive guide.

I extend my heartfelt thanks to the experts and professionals in the field of skincare, whose valuable knowledge and insights have greatly contributed to the content of this book. Your expertise and dedication to promoting natural and sustainable skincare practices have been invaluable in providing accurate and reliable information.

I am grateful to my family and friends for their unwavering support and encouragement throughout this writing journey. Your belief in my abilities and your constant motivation have been instrumental in bringing this book to fruition.

Lastly, I want to thank the readers for embarking on this journey of DIY natural skincare with me. I hope that the knowledge and insights shared in this book will empower you to take control of your skincare routine and discover the beauty of creating your own homemade products using natural ingredients.

Thank you all for your support, encouragement and contributions. This book would not have been possible without each and every one of you.

CHAPTER 1: UNDERSTANDING NATURAL SKINCARE

Definition and principles of natural skincare

Natural skincare refers to the practice of using ingredients derived from nature, such as plants, herbs, fruits, and oils, to care for and nourish the skin. It embraces a holistic approach that prioritizes the use of safe, non-toxic, and sustainable ingredients. The principles of natural skincare revolve around three key aspects: ingredient selection, formulation and environmental impact.

When it comes to ingredient selection, natural skincare avoids synthetic chemicals, harsh preservatives and artificial fragrances commonly found in commercial products. Instead, it focuses on utilizing plant-based ingredients known for their beneficial properties and compatibility with the skin. These ingredients are often rich in vitamins, antioxidants and essential fatty acids that promote skin health.

Formulation is another vital principle of natural skincare. It involves carefully blending natural ingredients to create effective and gentle products. Natural skincare formulations aim to strike a balance between providing nourishment, hydration and protection without compromising the skin's natural barrier function.

Lastly, natural skincare emphasizes environmental impact. It encourages the use of sustainably sourced ingredients, eco-friendly packaging and practices that minimize waste and pollution. By choosing natural skincare, individuals can reduce their carbon footprint and contribute to the preservation of the planet.

Natural skincare is characterized by ingredient transparency, gentle formulations, and a commitment to sustainability. It offers a holistic and conscious approach to skincare that promotes overall well-being while being kind to the environment.

Benefits of using natural ingredients

Using natural ingredients in skincare products offers a multitude of benefits for the skin and overall well-being. Here are several key advantages of incorporating natural ingredients into your skincare routine:

Gentle and non-irritating: Natural ingredients are typically milder and less likely to cause irritation or allergic reactions compared to synthetic ingredients commonly found in commercial products. This makes them suitable for individuals with sensitive skin or conditions like eczema or rosacea.

Nourishing and rejuvenating: Natural ingredients are often rich in vitamins, minerals, antioxidants, and essential fatty acids that provide essential nutrients to the skin. They help nourish, hydrate, and rejuvenate the skin, improving its overall health and appearance.

Effective without harmful chemicals: Natural ingredients offer effective skincare benefits without the use of potentially harmful chemicals such as parabens, sulfates, phthalates and synthetic fragrances. They provide a safer alternative for long-term skincare routines.

Compatibility with the skin: Natural ingredients are generally more compatible with the skin's natural biology. Their molecular structure is often similar to the skin's own components, allowing for better absorption and utilization of their beneficial properties.

Anti-inflammatory and soothing: Many natural ingredients possess anti-inflammatory properties, helping to calm and soothe irritated or inflamed skin. They can alleviate redness, itchiness and other signs of skin irritation.

Environmental sustainability: Using natural ingredients supports sustainable practices by reducing reliance on synthetic chemicals and minimizing environmental impact. Natural ingredients are often biodegradable, and their cultivation promotes biodiversity and reduces pollution.

The benefits of using natural ingredients in skincare products extend beyond skin health. They offer gentler, nourishing, and effective solutions while promoting sustainability and minimizing the risks associated with synthetic chemicals. Incorporating natural ingredients into your skincare routine allows for a more holistic approach to overall well-being.

Common harmful ingredients to avoid

When it comes to skincare products, it's essential to be aware of common harmful ingredients that should be avoided. These ingredients have been linked to various health concerns and can be detrimental to both your skin and overall well-being. Here are some common harmful ingredients to steer clear of:

Parabens: Widely used as preservatives, parabens have been associated with hormone disruption and potential links to breast cancer.

Sulfates: Sodium lauryl sulfate (SLS) and sodium laureth sulfate (SLES) are foaming agents that can strip the skin of its natural oils, leading to dryness and irritation.

Phthalates: Often found in fragrances, phthalates are known endocrine disruptors and have been linked to reproductive issues.

Synthetic Fragrances: Synthetic fragrances can cause skin irritation and allergic reactions in sensitive individuals. Look for products that use natural essential oils for fragrance.

Formaldehyde: Formaldehyde and formaldehyde-releasing preservatives (such as DMDM hydantoin and imidazolidinyl urea) can be skin irritants and have been classified as carcinogens.

Mineral Oil: Derived from petroleum, mineral oil can clog pores and create a barrier on the skin, preventing it from breathing and potentially leading to acne.

Synthetic Colors: Artificial colors like FD&C dyes are derived from coal tar and can cause skin sensitivity and irritation.

By avoiding these harmful ingredients and opting for natural and safer alternatives, you can make more informed choices about the products you use, reduce the risk of adverse reactions, and prioritize the health and well-being of your skin.

CHAPTER 2: GETTING STARTED WITH DIY SKINCARE

Essential tools and equipment

Having the right tools and equipment is crucial when it comes to creating DIY natural skincare products. Here are some essential items that can help you in your skincare formulation process:

Measuring Tools: Accurate measurements are essential for creating effective and safe skincare products. Invest in measuring spoons, graduated cylinders, or digital scales to ensure precise ingredient ratios.

Mixing Bowls and Utensils: Use glass or stainless steel bowls and utensils for mixing your ingredients.

These materials are non-reactive and easy to clean, ensuring there is no cross-contamination between different ingredients.

Double Boiler or Heatproof Container: A double boiler or heatproof container is necessary for gently heating ingredients that require melting or combining. It helps prevent direct heat exposure and maintains ingredient integrity.

Whisk or Hand Blender: Whisks or hand blenders are useful for emulsifying ingredients, ensuring proper blending and consistency in your formulations.

Sterilized Containers: Proper storage is essential to maintain the integrity and shelf life of your skincare products. Use sterilized glass or PET plastic containers with airtight lids to prevent contamination and prolong product freshness.

Pipettes or Droppers: Pipettes or droppers are handy tools for accurately measuring and dispensing small amounts of liquid ingredients like essential oils or carrier oils.

Labels and Markers: Labeling your skincare products is essential for easy identification and proper usage. Use waterproof labels and permanent markers to indicate the product name, ingredients, and date of creation.

Remember to maintain good hygiene practices by cleaning your tools and equipment before and after each use. This ensures the safety and effectiveness of your DIY skincare products. Having these essential tools and equipment will make your DIY skincare journey more organized, efficient, and enjoyable.

Importance of proper hygiene and safety measures

Proper hygiene and safety measures are of utmost importance when engaging in DIY skincare. Here's why:

Avoid Contamination: Maintaining cleanliness throughout the process is crucial to prevent contamination of your skincare products. Clean and disinfect your tools, containers, and work surfaces before and after use. This helps eliminate bacteria, mold and other microorganisms that can compromise the safety and effectiveness of your products.

Prevent Cross-Contamination: Cross-contamination can occur when different ingredients come into contact with one another, leading to unexpected reactions or spoilage. Use separate utensils and containers for each ingredient and ensure they are thoroughly cleaned between uses to prevent cross-contamination.

Ensure Product Safety: Proper hygiene measures help ensure the safety of your skincare products. By following good practices, you reduce the risk of bacterial growth, mold or other pathogens that could potentially harm your skin.

Protect Skin Health: Maintaining hygiene is not only about the safety of your products but also about protecting your skin. Working with clean tools and equipment reduces the likelihood of introducing irritants or harmful substances onto your skin, minimizing the risk of adverse reactions or skin infections.

Extend Shelf Life: Adhering to proper hygiene practices can help extend the shelf life of your DIY skincare products. By minimizing the introduction of contaminants, you improve the stability and longevity of your creations, ensuring they remain safe and effective for a longer period.

Personal Safety: Safety measures, such as wearing gloves when handling potentially irritating or harmful ingredients, protect you from direct contact and potential skin sensitivities or allergies. Additionally, be cautious when using heat or working with potentially hazardous substances, following appropriate safety guidelines to avoid accidents or burns.

By prioritizing proper hygiene and safety measures, you create a safe and clean environment for DIY skincare, ensuring the integrity and effectiveness of your products while safeguarding your skin and overall well-being.

Tips for sourcing high-quality natural ingredients

When sourcing high-quality natural ingredients for your DIY skincare creations, it's important to consider several factors to ensure their efficacy and safety. Here are some helpful tips:

Research and Select Reputable Suppliers: Take the time to research and choose reputable suppliers known for their commitment to quality and sustainability. Look for suppliers that provide information on the sourcing, extraction methods and certifications of their ingredients.

Choose Organic and Certified Ingredients: Opt for organic ingredients whenever possible. Organic certification ensures that the ingredients are free from synthetic pesticides, herbicides and genetic modifications. Look for certifications such as USDA Organic, Ecocert or COSMOS Organic.

Consider Extraction Methods: Pay attention to the extraction methods used to obtain the natural ingredients. Cold-pressed or steam-distilled methods are preferred as they preserve the integrity and beneficial properties of the ingredients.

Check for Purity: Ensure that the ingredients you choose are pure and free from additives, fillers or synthetic components. Read ingredient labels and avoid products that contain unnecessary additives or preservatives.

Check for Freshness: Natural ingredients have a limited shelf life. When purchasing, check the expiration or best-before dates to ensure freshness. Buying in smaller quantities can help prevent ingredient spoilage or degradation.

Consider Sustainable and Ethical Practices: Look for suppliers that prioritize sustainable practices, fair trade and ethical sourcing. This ensures that the ingredients are obtained in an environmentally and socially responsible manner.

Patch Test and Monitor Results: When introducing new ingredients to your skincare routine, it's crucial to conduct a patch test on a small area of your skin. This helps identify any potential allergies or sensitivities. Monitor your skin's response to ensure compatibility and desired results.

By following these tips, you can source high-quality natural ingredients for your DIY skincare products, ensuring their effectiveness, safety, and alignment with your values of sustainability and ethical practices.

CHAPTER 3: KEY INGREDIENTS FOR DIY SKINCARE

Overview of beneficial natural ingredients

A wide array of beneficial natural ingredients derived from plants, fruits, and oils can provide a wealth of advantages when incorporated into DIY skincare products. Each ingredient possesses unique properties that contribute to the overall health and appearance of the skin.

These natural ingredients offer a variety of benefits, including moisturizing, soothing, healing, and rejuvenating properties. They are rich in vitamins, antioxidants, essential fatty acids and other nourishing compounds that promote skin health.

From aloe vera's soothing and hydrating properties to jojoba oil's balancing and moisturizing effects, these natural ingredients address various skincare concerns. Rosehip seed oil aids in skin regeneration and improves the appearance of scars and wrinkles. Green tea extract provides antioxidant protection and reduces inflammation. Shea butter offers intense moisture and improves skin elasticity. Tea tree oil combats acne and soothes irritations, while chamomile extract calms sensitive skin.

Incorporating these natural ingredients into DIY skincare products allows individuals to harness their specific advantages and create personalized formulations. By utilizing nature's bounty, individuals can enhance their skincare routines and enjoy the numerous benefits these ingredients have to offer.

Properties and benefits of each ingredient

Each natural ingredient used in DIY skincare products possesses unique properties and offers a range of benefits for the skin. Here's a closer look at some key ingredients and their specific advantages:

Aloe Vera: Known for its soothing and hydrating properties, aloe vera helps calm inflammation, reduce redness, and promote healing. It moisturizes the skin without clogging pores, making it suitable for all skin types.

Jojoba Oil: With a composition similar to the skin's natural sebum, jojoba oil helps balance oil production, moisturize the skin, and maintain its elasticity. It is non-greasy and easily absorbed, making it an excellent choice for both dry and oily skin.

Rosehip Seed Oil: Packed with vitamins A, C, and E, antioxidants, and essential fatty acids, rosehip seed oil promotes skin regeneration, reduces the appearance of scars and wrinkles, and improves skin tone and texture. It also hydrates and nourishes the skin, leaving it radiant and rejuvenated.

Green Tea Extract: Rich in antioxidants, green tea extract helps protect the skin from free radical damage, reduces inflammation, and may assist in preventing premature aging. It can also improve skin texture, tone and clarity.

Shea Butter: With its high concentration of fatty acids and vitamins, shea butter provides intense moisture and nourishment to the skin. It helps soothe dryness, soften rough patches, and improve skin elasticity, making it an excellent choice for dry and mature skin.

Tea Tree Oil: Known for its antimicrobial and anti-inflammatory properties, tea tree oil helps combat acne, reduce redness and soothe skin irritations. It has natural antibacterial properties that help control oil production and keep the skin clear and balanced.

Chamomile Extract: Chamomile extract has anti-inflammatory properties, making it beneficial for soothing sensitive or irritated skin. It can calm redness, alleviate itching and dryness and promote overall skin health.

Understanding the properties and benefits of each natural ingredient allows for informed choices in formulating DIY skincare products. By utilizing these ingredients, individuals can harness their specific advantages and create personalized skincare routines to address various skin concerns effectively.

Where to find and how to store them

When it comes to finding and storing natural ingredients for DIY skincare, there are several options and considerations to keep in mind.

Local Stores: Many natural ingredients can be found at local health food stores, herbal shops, or specialty stores that focus on natural and organic products. These stores often carry a wide range of essential oils, carrier oils, herbal extracts and other natural skincare ingredients.

Online Retailers: Numerous online retailers specialize in natural ingredients for skincare. They offer a wide selection and convenient delivery options, making it easy to access a variety of ingredients from the comfort of your home. Look for reputable online stores that provide detailed product information and customer reviews.

Farmer's Markets: Farmer's markets are great places to find locally sourced natural ingredients. You can often find fresh herbs, oils, and other botanical ingredients directly from farmers and local producers. This supports local businesses and ensures the freshness and quality of the ingredients.

DIY Suppliers: Some suppliers specifically cater to DIY skincare enthusiasts and offer a wide range of natural ingredients, packaging materials and tools. These suppliers often have comprehensive ingredient lists, product descriptions and helpful tips for formulation.

When it comes to storing natural ingredients, proper storage helps maintain their potency and prolong their shelf life:

Cool and Dark: Store ingredients in cool, dark places, away from direct sunlight and heat. Exposure to light, heat, and air can degrade the quality and efficacy of the ingredients.

Airtight Containers: Transfer ingredients into airtight containers, preferably made of glass or opaque plastic, to protect them from air and moisture. Ensure the containers are clean and dry before storing the ingredients.

Labeling: Label each ingredient with its name, date of purchase, and expiration date, if applicable. This helps you keep track of freshness and ensures you use them within their recommended timeline.

By sourcing ingredients from reputable sources and storing them properly, you can maintain their quality, potency, and effectiveness, ensuring optimal results when creating your DIY skincare products.

CHAPTER 4: BASIC DIY SKIN-CARE RECIPES

CLEANSERS AND TONERS

DIY cleansers and toners are homemade skincare products that can be crafted using natural ingredients readily available at home or easily sourced from local stores. These DIY formulations offer several advantages, such as customization, affordability, and the ability to control the ingredients used.

DIY cleansers are designed to remove dirt, impurities, and excess oil from the skin, leaving it clean and refreshed. They can be tailored to specific skin types and concerns by adjusting the ingredients. Common ingredients used in DIY cleansers include honey, yogurt, oils, fruits, and gentle exfoliants like oatmeal or sugar.

DIY toners, on the other hand, are used after cleansing to balance the skin's pH, tighten pores, and prepare the skin for moisturization. Toners can help soothe, hydrate, or clarify the skin depending on the chosen ingredients. Popular choices include witch hazel, rosewater, apple cider vinegar and herbal infusions.

Creating DIY cleansers and toners allows individuals to have complete control over the ingredients, ensuring they are free from harsh chemicals and artificial additives that may be present in commercial products. Additionally, DIY formulations can be cost-effective and environmentally friendly.

It's important to note that everyone's skin is unique, and what works for one person may not work for another. It's always recommended to do a patch test before using any new DIY skincare product and to consult with a dermatologist if you have any specific skin concerns or sensitivities.

Ingredients:

- 1 tbsp raw honey (preferably organic)
- 1 tbsp liquid castile soap
- 2 tbsp distilled water
- 1 tsp jojoba oil (or any carrier oil of your choice)
- 5 drops lavender essential oil (optional)

Instructions:

1. In a small bowl, combine 1 tbsp raw honey, 1 tbsp liquid castile soap, and 2 tbsp distilled water.
2. Add 1 tsp jojoba oil and 5 drops of lavender essential oil (optional).
3. Mix the ingredients well until they are thoroughly combined.
4. Transfer the mixture to a clean bottle or container for storage.

Usage:

1. Wet your face with water.
2. Take a small amount of the honey cleansing face wash in your palm.
3. Gently massage the cleanser onto your face using circular motions for about a minute.
4. Rinse off thoroughly with lukewarm water.
5. Pat dry and follow up with your regular skincare routine.

Storage:

- Store the honey cleansing face wash in a sealed container at room temperature.
- Use within 2-3 months.
- Keep away from direct sunlight and heat sources.
- Before each use, give the cleanser a quick shake to ensure proper blending.

Note: Perform a patch test before using, especially if you have sensitive skin. Discontinue if any irritation occurs.

Ingredients:

- 2 tbsp oats
- 1/2 cup milk (dairy or plant-based)
- 1 tsp honey (optional)
- 2-3 drops of essential oil (optional)

Instructions:

1. Grind 2 tbsp oats into a fine powder.
2. In a small saucepan, heat 1/2 cup milk until warm (not boiling).
3. Add the ground oats to the warm milk and let it sit for 5 minutes.
4. Strain the mixture to remove any larger oat particles.
5. If desired, add 1 tsp honey and 2-3 drops of essential oil for added benefits and fragrance. Mix well.

Usage:

1. Apply the cleansing milk to your damp face, gently massaging in circular motions.
2. Rinse off with warm water.
3. Pat dry and follow up with your regular skincare routine.

Storage:

- Store any leftover cleansing milk in a sealed container in the refrigerator.
- Use within 3-4 days.

- Before each use, shake well to ensure proper mixing.

Note: Perform a patch test before using. Discontinue if
any irritation occurs.

Ingredients:

- 1 green tea bag
- 1/2 cup hot water
- 2 tbsp liquid castile soap
- 1 tsp olive oil (or any carrier oil of your choice)
- 2-3 drops of essential oil (optional)

Instructions:

1. Steep 1 green tea bag in 1/2 cup of hot water for 5-10 minutes.
2. Remove the tea bag and let the green tea cool to room temperature.
3. In a small bowl, combine 2 tbsp liquid castile soap, 1 tsp olive oil, and 2-3 drops of essential oil (optional). Mix well.
4. Add the cooled green tea to the mixture and stir until everything is well combined.
5. Transfer the mixture to a bottle or container for storage.

Usage:

1. Wet your face with water.
2. Apply a small amount of the green tea facial cleanser to your palm.
3. Gently massage the cleanser onto your face in circular motions for about a minute.
4. Rinse off thoroughly with water.

5. Pat dry and follow up with your regular skincare routine.

Storage:

- Store the green tea facial cleanser in a sealed container at room temperature.
- Use within 2-3 weeks.
- Shake well before each use to ensure proper mixing.

Note: Perform a patch test before using. Discontinue if any irritation occurs.

Ingredients:

- 1/2 cucumber
- 2 tbsp plain yogurt (unsweetened)
- 1 tbsp aloe vera gel
- 1 tsp lemon juice (optional)
- 2-3 drops of essential oil (optional)

Instructions:

1. Peel and chop half a cucumber into small pieces.
2. Place the chopped cucumber in a blender or food processor and blend until smooth.
3. In a small bowl, combine 2 tbsp plain yogurt, 1 tbsp aloe vera gel, and 1 tsp lemon juice (optional).
4. Add the blended cucumber to the mixture and stir until well mixed.
5. If desired, add 2-3 drops of essential oil for added benefits and fragrance. Mix well.
6. Transfer the mixture to a bottle or container for storage.

Usage:

1. Wet your face with water.
2. Apply a small amount of the yogurt and cucumber cleanser to your palm.
3. Gently massage the cleanser onto your face in circular motions for about a minute.
4. Rinse off thoroughly with water.

5. Pat dry and follow up with your regular skincare routine.

Storage:

- Store the yogurt and cucumber cleanser in a sealed container in the refrigerator.
- Use within 3-4 days.
- Before each use, shake well to ensure proper mixing.

Note: Perform a patch test before using. Discontinue if any irritation occurs.

Ingredients:

- 2 tbsp coconut oil (organic, unrefined)
- 1 tbsp honey (raw, optional)
- 2-3 drops of essential oil (optional)

Instructions:

1. In a small bowl, measure 2 tbsp of coconut oil.
2. If desired, add 1 tbsp of raw honey to the bowl. Mix well.
3. If using, add 2-3 drops of essential oil for added benefits and fragrance. Mix well.
4. The coconut oil may solidify, so warm the mixture slightly to melt it if needed.
5. Transfer the mixture to a jar or container for storage.

Usage:

1. Take a small amount of the coconut oil cleanser in your hands.
2. Gently massage it onto your dry face, using circular motions to dissolve makeup and impurities.
3. Wet a washcloth with warm water and place it over your face to steam for a few seconds.
4. Wipe away the cleanser and rinse the washcloth as needed.
5. Rinse your face with warm water to remove any residue.

6. Pat dry and follow up with your regular skincare routine.

Storage:

- Store the coconut oil cleanser in a sealed container at room temperature.
- It may solidify in cooler temperatures, but it will melt upon contact with warm skin.
- Use within 3-4 months.
- Before each use, mix well if any separation occurs.

Note: Perform a patch test before using, especially if you have oily or acne-prone skin. Discontinue if any irritation occurs.

Ingredients:

- 1 tbsp honey (raw, preferably organic)
- 1 tsp lemon juice (freshly squeezed)
- 1 tbsp water (filtered, if possible)

Instructions:

1. In a small bowl, combine 1 tbsp of honey, 1 tsp of lemon juice, and 1 tbsp of water.
2. Stir the mixture well until all the ingredients are thoroughly blended.
3. If desired, warm the mixture slightly to help the honey dissolve.
4. Transfer the mixture to a small, clean container for storage.

Usage:

1. Wet your face with water.
2. Take a small amount of the honey and lemon cleanser in your palm.
3. Gently massage the cleanser onto your face using circular motions for about a minute.
4. Rinse off thoroughly with lukewarm water.
5. Pat dry and follow up with your regular skincare routine.

Storage:

- Store the honey and lemon cleanser in a sealed container at room temperature.
- Use within 1-2 weeks.

- Keep away from direct sunlight and heat sources.
- Before each use, give the cleanser a quick stir to ensure proper blending.

Note: Perform a patch test before using, especially if you have sensitive skin. Discontinue if any irritation occurs.

Ingredients:

- 1/2 cucumber
- 1/4 cup fresh mint leaves
- 1 tbsp witch hazel
- 1 tbsp lemon juice (freshly squeezed)
- 1 tbsp water (filtered, if possible)

Instructions:

1. Peel and chop half a cucumber into small pieces.
2. In a blender or food processor, combine the chopped cucumber, fresh mint leaves, witch hazel, lemon juice, and water.
3. Blend the ingredients until you have a smooth, liquid consistency.
4. Transfer the mixture to a small, clean container for storage.

Usage:

1. Wet your face with water.
2. Take a small amount of the cucumber and mint cleanser in your palm.
3. Gently massage the cleanser onto your face using circular motions for about a minute.
4. Rinse off thoroughly with lukewarm water.
5. Pat dry and follow up with your regular skincare routine.

Storage:

- Store the cucumber and mint cleanser in a sealed container in the refrigerator.
- Use within 1-2 weeks.
- Keep away from direct sunlight and heat sources.
- Before each use, give the cleanser a quick shake or stir to ensure proper blending.

Note: Perform a patch test before using, especially if you have sensitive skin. Discontinue if any irritation occurs.

Ingredients:
- 2 tbsp plain yogurt (unsweetened)
- 1/2 tsp turmeric powder
- 1 tsp honey (raw, optional)

Instructions:
1. In a small bowl, combine 2 tbsp of plain yogurt and 1/2 tsp of turmeric powder.
2. If desired, add 1 tsp of raw honey for added benefits and moisturization.
3. Mix the ingredients well until they form a smooth paste.
4. Transfer the mixture to a clean container for storage.

Usage:
1. Wet your face with water.
2. Take a small amount of the yogurt and turmeric cleanser in your palm.
3. Gently massage the cleanser onto your face using circular motions for about a minute.
4. Allow the cleanser to sit on your skin for an additional minute to benefit from the turmeric.
5. Rinse off thoroughly with lukewarm water.
6. Pat dry and follow up with your regular skincare routine.

Storage:

- Store the yogurt and turmeric cleanser in a sealed container in the refrigerator.
- Use within 1-2 weeks.
- Keep away from direct sunlight and heat sources.
- Before each use, give the cleanser a quick stir to ensure proper blending.

Note: Turmeric may leave a temporary yellow tint on the skin, so be cautious when using white towels or clothing. Perform a patch test before using, especially if you have sensitive or reactive skin. Discontinue if any irritation occurs.

Ingredients:

- 1/4 cup coconut milk (canned or homemade)
- 2 tbsp aloe vera gel (pure and organic)
- 1 tsp almond oil (or any carrier oil of your choice)
- 5 drops of tea tree essential oil (optional)

Instructions:

1. In a small bowl, combine 1/4 cup of coconut milk and 2 tbsp of aloe vera gel.
2. Add 1 tsp of almond oil and 5 drops of tea tree essential oil (optional).
3. Mix the ingredients well until they are thoroughly combined.
4. Transfer the mixture to a clean bottle or container for storage.

Usage:

1. Wet your face with water.
2. Take a small amount of the coconut milk and aloe vera cleanser in your palm.
3. Gently massage the cleanser onto your face using circular motions for about a minute.
4. Rinse off thoroughly with lukewarm water.
5. Pat dry and follow up with your regular skincare routine.

Storage:

- Store the coconut milk and aloe vera cleanser in a sealed container in the refrigerator.

- Use within 1-2 weeks.

- Keep away from direct sunlight and heat sources.

- Before each use, give the cleanser a quick shake or stir to ensure proper blending.

Note: Perform a patch test before using, especially if you have sensitive skin. Discontinue if any irritation occurs.

Ingredients:

- 1/2 ripe papaya
- 1 tbsp honey (raw, preferably organic)
- 1 tsp lemon juice (freshly squeezed)

Instructions:

1. Peel the papaya and remove the seeds.
2. Cut the papaya into small pieces and place them in a blender or food processor.
3. Blend the papaya until you have a smooth puree.
4. In a small bowl, combine 1/4 cup of the papaya puree with 1 tbsp of honey and 1 tsp of lemon juice.
5. Mix the ingredients well until they form a smooth mixture.
6. Transfer the mixture to a clean container for storage.

Usage:

1. Wet your face with water.
2. Take a small amount of the papaya cleanser in your palm.
3. Gently massage the cleanser onto your face using circular motions for about a minute.
4. Rinse off thoroughly with lukewarm water.
5. Pat dry and follow up with your regular skincare routine.

Storage:

- Store the papaya cleanser in a sealed container in the refrigerator.
- Use within 1 week.
- Keep away from direct sunlight and heat sources.
- Before each use, give the cleanser a quick stir to ensure proper blending.

Note: Papaya contains natural enzymes that can exfoliate the skin. Perform a patch test before using, especially if you have sensitive skin. Discontinue if any irritation occurs.

Ingredients:

- 1/2 ripe papaya
- 1 tbsp honey (raw, preferably organic)
- 1 tsp lemon juice (freshly squeezed)

Instructions:

1. Peel the papaya and remove the seeds.
2. Cut the papaya into small pieces and place them in a blender or food processor.
3. Blend the papaya until you have a smooth puree.
4. In a small bowl, combine 1/4 cup of the papaya puree with 1 tbsp of honey and 1 tsp of lemon juice.
5. Mix the ingredients well until they form a smooth mixture.
6. Transfer the mixture to a clean container for storage.

Usage:

1. Wet your face with water.
2. Take a small amount of the papaya cleanser in your palm.
3. Gently massage the cleanser onto your face using circular motions for about a minute.
4. Rinse off thoroughly with lukewarm water.
5. Pat dry and follow up with your regular skincare routine.

Storage:

- Store the papaya cleanser in a sealed container in the refrigerator.
- Use within 1 week.
- Keep away from direct sunlight and heat sources.
- Before each use, give the cleanser a quick stir to ensure proper blending.

Note: Papaya contains natural enzymes that can exfoliate the skin. Perform a patch test before using, especially if you have sensitive skin. Discontinue if any irritation occurs.

Ingredients:

- 1/2 cucumber
- 1/4 cup witch hazel
- 1/4 cup water (filtered)
- 5 drops lavender essential oil (optional)

Instructions:

1. Peel the cucumber and chop it into small pieces.
2. Place the cucumber pieces in a blender or food processor and blend until smooth.
3. Strain the cucumber puree using a fine-mesh sieve to extract the juice.
4. In a small bottle or container, combine 1/4 cup of witch hazel, 1/4 cup of filtered water, and the cucumber juice.
5. If desired, add 5 drops of lavender essential oil for added soothing properties.
6. Close the bottle or container tightly and shake well to mix the ingredients.

Usage:

1. After cleansing your face, pour a small amount of the cucumber and witch hazel toner onto a cotton pad or ball.
2. Gently swipe the cotton pad across your face, avoiding the eye area.
3. Allow the toner to air dry on your skin.
4. Follow up with your regular moisturizer or serum.

Storage:

- Store the cucumber and witch hazel toner in a sealed bottle or container in the refrigerator.
- Use within 1-2 weeks.
- Keep away from direct sunlight and heat sources.
- Shake well before each use to ensure proper blending.

Note: Perform a patch test before using, especially if you have sensitive skin. Discontinue if any irritation occurs.

Ingredients:

- 1/2 cup rosewater
- 1/4 cup aloe vera gel
- 1 tsp glycerin (optional)
- 5 drops rose essential oil (optional)

Instructions:

1. In a small bottle or container, combine 1/2 cup of rosewater and 1/4 cup of aloe vera gel.
2. If desired, add 1 tsp of glycerin for added moisturization.
3. If using, add 5 drops of rose essential oil for a pleasant fragrance.
4. Close the bottle or container tightly and shake well to mix the ingredients.

Usage:

1. After cleansing your face, pour a small amount of the rosewater and aloe vera toner onto a cotton pad or ball.
2. Gently swipe the cotton pad across your face, avoiding the eye area.
3. Allow the toner to air dry on your skin.
4. Follow up with your regular moisturizer or serum.

Storage:

- Store the rosewater and aloe vera toner in a sealed bottle or container at room temperature.
- Use within 1-2 months.

- Keep away from direct sunlight and heat sources.
- Shake well before each use to ensure proper blending.

Note: Perform a patch test before using, especially if you have sensitive skin. Discontinue if any irritation occurs.

Ingredients:

- 1 green tea bag
- 1/2 cup hot water
- 1/4 cup witch hazel
- 5 drops tea tree essential oil (optional)

Instructions:

1. Steep 1 green tea bag in 1/2 cup of hot water for 5-10 minutes.
2. Remove the tea bag and let the green tea cool to room temperature.
3. In a small bottle or container, combine 1/4 cup of witch hazel and the cooled green tea.
4. If desired, add 5 drops of tea tree essential oil for added antibacterial properties.
- Close the bottle or container tightly and shake well to mix the ingredients.

Usage:

1. After cleansing your face, pour a small amount of the green tea toner onto a cotton pad or ball.
2. Gently swipe the cotton pad across your face, avoiding the eye area.
3. Allow the toner to air dry on your skin.
4. Follow up with your regular moisturizer or serum.

Storage:

- Store the green tea toner in a sealed bottle or container at room temperature.

- Use within 1-2 weeks.
- Keep away from direct sunlight and heat sources.
- Shake well before each use to ensure proper blending.

Note: Perform a patch test before using, especially if you have sensitive skin. Discontinue if any irritation occurs.

Ingredients:

- 1 chamomile tea bag
- 1/2 cup hot water
- 1/4 cup witch hazel

Instructions:

1. Steep 1 chamomile tea bag in 1/2 cup of hot water for 5-10 minutes.
2. Remove the tea bag and let the chamomile tea cool to room temperature.
3. In a small bottle or container, combine 1/4 cup of witch hazel and the cooled chamomile tea.
4. Close the bottle or container tightly and shake well to mix the ingredients.

Usage:

1. After cleansing your face, pour a small amount of the chamomile toner onto a cotton pad or ball.
2. Gently swipe the cotton pad across your face, avoiding the eye area.
3. Allow the toner to air dry on your skin.
4. Follow up with your regular moisturizer or serum.

Storage:

- Store the chamomile toner in a sealed bottle or container at room temperature.
- Use within 1-2 weeks.
- Keep away from direct sunlight and heat sources.

- Shake well before each use to ensure proper blending.

Note: Chamomile is generally gentle on the skin, but perform a patch test before using, especially if you have sensitive skin. Discontinue if any irritation occurs.

Ingredients:

- 1/2 cup water (filtered)
- 1/4 cup witch hazel
- 10 drops lavender essential oil

Instructions:

1. In a small bottle or container, combine 1/2 cup of filtered water and 1/4 cup of witch hazel.
2. Add 10 drops of lavender essential oil to the mixture.
3. Close the bottle or container tightly and shake well to mix the ingredients.

Usage:

1. After cleansing your face, pour a small amount of the lavender toner onto a cotton pad or ball.
2. Gently swipe the cotton pad across your face, avoiding the eye area.
3. Allow the toner to air dry on your skin.
4. Follow up with your regular moisturizer or serum.

Storage:

- Store the lavender toner in a sealed bottle or container at room temperature.
- Use within 1-2 months.
- Keep away from direct sunlight and heat sources.
- Shake well before each use to ensure proper blending.

Note: Lavender essential oil may cause irritation in some individuals. Perform a patch test before using, especially if you have sensitive skin. Discontinue if any irritation occurs.

Ingredients:

- 1 cup water (filtered)
- 1/4 cup fresh mint leaves
- 1/4 cup witch hazel

Instructions:

1. In a small saucepan, bring 1 cup of filtered water to a boil.
2. Add 1/4 cup of fresh mint leaves to the boiling water and let it simmer for 5 minutes.
3. Remove the saucepan from heat and allow the mint water to cool down.
4. Strain the mint water using a fine-mesh sieve to remove the mint leaves.
5. In a small bottle or container, combine 1/4 cup of the mint water with 1/4 cup of witch hazel.
6. Close the bottle or container tightly and shake well to mix the ingredients.

Usage:

1. After cleansing your face, pour a small amount of the mint toner onto a cotton pad or ball.
2. Gently swipe the cotton pad across your face, avoiding the eye area.
3. Allow the toner to air dry on your skin.
4. Follow up with your regular moisturizer or serum.

Storage:

- Store the mint toner in a sealed bottle or container in the refrigerator.
- Use within 1-2 weeks.
- Keep away from direct sunlight and heat sources.
- Shake well before each use to ensure proper blending.

Note: Mint may cause irritation in some individuals, especially those with sensitive skin. Perform a patch test before using. Discontinue if any irritation occurs.

MOISTURIZERS AND SERUMS

DIY skincare allows you to create your own moisturizers and serums tailored to your skin's specific needs. Moisturizers are crucial for hydrating and nourishing the skin, while serums provide targeted treatments for various concerns. By making these products yourself, you have control over the ingredients, ensuring they are natural, high-quality and suited to your skin type.

When it comes to DIY moisturizers, you can choose from a variety of ingredients such as oils, butters and botanical extracts. Carrier oils like jojoba, almond, or coconut oil are popular choices as they provide deep hydration and can be easily customized with essential oils or herbal infusions. Butters like shea or cocoa butter offer rich emollient properties, ideal for dry or mature skin. You can also incorporate humectants like glycerin or hyaluronic acid to attract and retain moisture in the skin.

DIY serums are highly concentrated formulations designed to address specific skin concerns. Vitamin C serums are popular for brightening and evening out skin tone, while hyaluronic acid serums provide intense hydration. You can also create serums targeting acne, aging, or hyperpigmentation by incorporating ingredients like tea tree oil, retinol, or niacinamide. Aloe vera gel or witch hazel can serve as excellent base ingredients for serums, providing soothing and toning properties.

When creating DIY moisturizers and serums, it's essential to maintain proper hygiene and storage. Use clean utensils and containers to prevent contamination, and store your products in dark glass bottles or jars to protect them from light and air. Keep in mind that homemade skincare products may have a shorter shelf life compared to commercial ones, so it's important to monitor their freshness and discard any products that show signs of spoilage.

Before incorporating any new DIY moisturizers or serums into your skincare routine, it's recommended to conduct a patch test to ensure compatibility with your skin. Apply a small amount to a discreet area and monitor for any adverse reactions. Additionally, it's wise to consult a dermatologist or skincare professional if you have specific skin conditions or concerns to ensure the safety and effectiveness of your homemade products.

DIY moisturizers and serums offer a personalized and cost-effective approach to skincare. By exploring different ingredients and formulations, you can create products that not only nourish and protect your skin but also provide a luxurious and enjoyable experience. Whether you're looking for intense hydration, anti-aging benefits, or targeted treatments, DIY skincare allows you to take charge of your beauty routine and unleash your creativity.

Ingredients:
- Organic, unrefined coconut oil

Instructions:
1. Take a small amount of organic, unrefined coconut oil in your palm.
2. Rub your palms together to warm up the oil and melt it.
3. Gently apply the melted coconut oil to your skin.
4. Massage the oil into your skin until it is fully absorbed.
5. Adjust the amount of coconut oil according to your skin's needs.

Usage:
1. Apply the coconut oil moisturizer to your skin after cleansing.
2. Use it daily or as needed to keep your skin hydrated.
3. Focus on dry areas or areas that need extra moisture.

Storage:
- Store the coconut oil in a cool, dry place at room temperature.
- Keep away from direct sunlight and heat sources.
- Coconut oil has a long shelf life and can be stored for several months.

Note: Coconut oil is generally safe for most skin types, but it may not be suitable for everyone, especially those with oily or acne-prone skin. Perform a patch test before using. Discontinue if any irritation occurs.

Ingredients:

- 1/2 cup shea butter (raw, unrefined)
- Optional: a few drops of essential oil (such as lavender or rose)

Instructions:

1. In a double boiler, melt 1/2 cup of raw, unrefined shea butter over low heat.
2. Once melted, remove from heat and let it cool for a few minutes.
3. Optional: Add a few drops of your preferred essential oil to the melted shea butter and stir well.
4. Transfer the mixture to a clean container or jar for storage.

Usage:

1. Take a small amount of the shea butter moisturizer with clean fingers.
2. Gently rub the shea butter between your palms to warm it up.
3. Apply the melted shea butter to your skin and massage it in until fully absorbed.
4. Adjust the amount of moisturizer according to your skin's needs.

Storage:

- Store the shea butter moisturizer in a cool, dry place at room temperature.
- Keep away from direct sunlight and heat sources.

- Shea butter has a long shelf life and can be stored for several months.

Note: Shea butter is generally safe for most skin types, but perform a patch test before using, especially if you have nut allergies or sensitive skin. Discontinue if any irritation occurs.

Ingredients:
- Pure aloe vera gel

Instructions:
1. Take a small amount of pure aloe vera gel in your palm.
2. Gently rub your palms together to warm up the gel.
3. Apply the aloe vera gel to your skin and massage it in until fully absorbed.
4. Adjust the amount of gel according to your skin's needs.

Usage:
1. Apply the aloe vera gel moisturizer to your skin after cleansing.
2. Use it daily or as needed to keep your skin hydrated.
3. Focus on dry areas or areas that need extra moisture.

Storage:
- Store the aloe vera gel in a sealed container in the refrigerator.
- Use within 2-3 weeks.
- Keep away from direct sunlight and heat sources.
- Aloe vera gel can spoil quickly, so it's important to check for any signs of mold or spoilage before each use.

Note: Aloe vera gel is generally safe for most skin types, but perform a patch test before using, especially if you have sensitive skin. Discontinue if any irritation occurs.

Ingredients:

- Raw honey

Instructions:

1. Take a small amount of raw honey in your palm.
2. Gently rub your palms together to warm up the honey.
3. Apply the honey to your skin and massage it in until fully absorbed.
4. Adjust the amount of honey according to your skin's needs.

Usage:

1. Apply the honey moisturizer to your skin after cleansing.
2. Use it daily or as needed to keep your skin hydrated.
3. Focus on dry areas or areas that need extra moisture.

Storage:

- Store the raw honey in a cool, dry place at room temperature.
- Keep away from direct sunlight and heat sources.
- Honey has a long shelf life and can be stored for several months.

Note: Honey is generally safe for most skin types, but perform a patch test before using, especially if you have al-

lergies or sensitive skin. Discontinue if any irritation occurs.

Ingredients:

- Extra virgin olive oil

Instructions:

1. Take a small amount of extra virgin olive oil in your palm.
2. Gently rub your palms together to warm up the oil.
3. Apply the olive oil to your skin and massage it in until fully absorbed.
4. Adjust the amount of oil according to your skin's needs.

Usage:

1. Apply the olive oil moisturizer to your skin after cleansing.
2. Use it daily or as needed to keep your skin hydrated.
3. Focus on dry areas or areas that need extra moisture.

Storage:

- Store the olive oil in a cool, dark place at room temperature.
- Keep away from direct sunlight and heat sources.
- Olive oil has a long shelf life and can be stored for several months.

Note: Olive oil is generally safe for most skin types, but it may not be suitable for everyone, especially those with oily or acne-prone skin. Perform a patch test before using. Discontinue if any irritation occurs.

Ingredients:

- 1/2 cup cocoa butter
- Optional: a few drops of essential oil (such as lavender or vanilla)

Instructions:

1. In a double boiler, melt 1/2 cup of cocoa butter over low heat until it becomes liquid.
2. Remove from heat and let it cool for a few minutes.
3. Optional: Add a few drops of your preferred essential oil to the melted cocoa butter and stir well.
4. Transfer the mixture to a clean container or jar for storage.

Usage:

1. Take a small amount of the cocoa butter moisturizer with clean fingers.
2. Gently rub the cocoa butter between your palms to warm it up.
3. Apply the melted cocoa butter to your skin and massage it in until fully absorbed.
4. Adjust the amount of moisturizer according to your skin's needs.

Storage:

- Store the cocoa butter moisturizer in a cool, dry place at room temperature.
- Keep away from direct sunlight and heat sources.

- Cocoa butter has a long shelf life and can be stored for several months.

Note: Cocoa butter is generally safe for most skin types, but perform a patch test before using, especially if you have sensitive skin or cocoa allergies. Discontinue if any irritation occurs.

Ingredients:

- 1 ripe avocado

Instructions:

1. Cut open a ripe avocado and scoop out the flesh into a bowl.
2. Mash the avocado until it becomes a smooth paste.
3. Optional: Add a teaspoon of honey or a few drops of olive oil for added moisturization.
4. Mix well to combine all the ingredients.

Usage:

1. Take a small amount of the avocado moisturizer with clean fingers.
2. Gently apply the avocado paste to your skin and massage it in until fully absorbed.
3. Adjust the amount of moisturizer according to your skin's needs.

Storage:

- Store the avocado moisturizer in a sealed container or jar in the refrigerator.
- Use within 2-3 days.
- Keep away from direct sunlight and heat sources.
- Avocado can spoil quickly, so it's important to check for any signs of spoilage before each use.

Note: Avocado is generally safe for most skin types, but perform a patch test before using, especially if you have avocado allergies or sensitive skin. Discontinue if any irritation occurs.

Ingredients:

- Jojoba oil

Instructions:

1. Take a small amount of jojoba oil in your palm.
2. Gently rub your palms together to warm up the oil.
3. Apply the jojoba oil to your skin and massage it in until fully absorbed.
4. Adjust the amount of oil according to your skin's needs.

Usage:

1. Apply the jojoba oil moisturizer to your skin after cleansing.
2. Use it daily or as needed to keep your skin hydrated.
3. Focus on dry areas or areas that need extra moisture.

Storage:

- Store the jojoba oil in a cool, dark place at room temperature.
- Keep away from direct sunlight and heat sources.
- Jojoba oil has a long shelf life and can be stored for several months.

Note: Jojoba oil is generally safe for most skin types, but perform a patch test before using, especially if you have nut allergies or sensitive skin. Discontinue if any irritation occurs.

Ingredients:

- Rosehip oil

Instructions:

1. Take a small amount of rosehip oil in your palm.
2. Gently rub your palms together to warm up the oil.
3. Apply the rosehip oil to your skin and massage it in until fully absorbed.
4. Adjust the amount of oil according to your skin's needs.

Usage:

1. Apply the rosehip oil moisturizer to your skin after cleansing.
2. Use it daily or as needed to keep your skin hydrated.
3. Focus on dry areas or areas that need extra moisture.

Storage:

- Store the rosehip oil in a cool, dark place at room temperature.
- Keep away from direct sunlight and heat sources.
- Rosehip oil has a long shelf life and can be stored for several months.

Note: Rosehip oil is generally safe for most skin types, but perform a patch test before using, especially if you have allergies or sensitive skin. Discontinue if any irritation occurs.

Ingredients:

- 1 small cucumber

Instructions:

1. Peel and chop a small cucumber into small pieces.
2. Blend the cucumber pieces in a blender or food processor until you have a smooth paste.
3. Optional: Strain the cucumber pulp to obtain a smoother consistency.
4. Transfer the cucumber paste to a clean container or jar for storage.

Usage:

1. Take a small amount of the cucumber moisturizer with clean fingers.
2. Gently apply the cucumber paste to your skin and massage it in until fully absorbed.
3. Adjust the amount of moisturizer according to your skin's needs.

Storage:

- Store the cucumber moisturizer in a sealed container or jar in the refrigerator.
- Use within 2-3 days.
- Keep away from direct sunlight and heat sources.
- Check for any signs of spoilage before each use.

Note: Cucumber is generally safe for most skin types, but perform a patch test before using, especially if you have cucumber allergies or sensitive skin. Discontinue if any irritation occurs.

Ingredients:

- 1 teaspoon vitamin C powder
- 1 tablespoon distilled water
- Optional: a few drops of vegetable glycerin or aloe vera gel

Instructions:

1. In a small bowl, combine 1 teaspoon of vitamin C powder with 1 tablespoon of distilled water.
2. Stir the mixture until the vitamin C powder is fully dissolved.
3. Optional: Add a few drops of vegetable glycerin or aloe vera gel to the mixture and stir well to combine.

Usage:

1. After cleansing your face, apply a small amount of the vitamin C serum to your skin.
2. Gently massage the serum into your skin until fully absorbed.
3. Allow the serum to dry before applying moisturizer or other skincare products.

Storage:

- Store the vitamin C serum in a small, dark-colored glass bottle with a dropper for easy application.
- Keep the bottle tightly sealed to prevent oxidation.
- Store in a cool, dark place, away from direct sunlight and heat sources.

- Use within 1-2 weeks for optimal freshness and potency.

Note: Vitamin C serums can be sensitizing for some individuals. If you experience any irritation or discomfort, discontinue use. It's recommended to perform a patch test before applying the serum to your face.

Ingredients:

- 1 tablespoon rosehip oil
- Optional: a few drops of vitamin E oil
- Optional: a drop or two of lavender or frankincense essential oil

Instructions:

1. In a small bottle or container, combine 1 tablespoon of rosehip oil with a few drops of vitamin E oil.
2. Optionally, add a drop or two of lavender or frankincense essential oil for added benefits.
3. Close the bottle or container tightly and shake well to mix the ingredients.

Usage:

1. After cleansing your face, apply a small amount of the rosehip oil serum to your skin.
2. Gently massage the serum into your skin until fully absorbed.
3. Allow the serum to dry before applying moisturizer or other skincare products.

Storage:

- Store the rosehip oil serum in a small, dark-colored glass bottle with a dropper for easy application.
- Keep the bottle tightly sealed to protect the oil from oxidation.

- Store in a cool, dark place, away from direct sunlight and heat sources.
- Use within 6-12 months for optimal freshness and potency.

Note: Rosehip oil is generally safe for most skin types, but perform a patch test before using, especially if you have sensitive skin or allergies. Discontinue use if any irritation occurs.

Ingredients:
- 1 tablespoon jojoba oil
- A few drops of frankincense essential oil
- Optional: a drop of geranium essential oil

Instructions:
1. In a small bottle or container, combine 1 tablespoon of jojoba oil with a few drops of frankincense essential oil.
2. Optionally, add a drop of geranium essential oil for a pleasant fragrance.
3. Close the bottle or container tightly and shake well to mix the ingredients.

Usage:
1. After cleansing your face, apply a small amount of the frankincense and jojoba serum to your skin.
2. Gently massage the serum into your skin until fully absorbed.
3. Allow the serum to dry before applying moisturizer or other skincare products.

Storage:
- Store the frankincense and jojoba serum in a small, dark-colored glass bottle with a dropper for easy application.
- Keep the bottle tightly sealed to protect the oils from oxidation.

- Store in a cool, dark place, away from direct sunlight and heat sources.
- Use within 6-12 months for optimal freshness and potency.

Note: Essential oils can cause skin irritation in some individuals. Perform a patch test before using, especially if you have sensitive skin or allergies. Discontinue use if any irritation occurs.

Ingredients:

- 1 tablespoon argan oil
- A few drops of rosehip oil
- Optional: a drop of ylang-ylang or lavender essential oil

Instructions:

1. In a small bottle or container, combine 1 tablespoon of argan oil with a few drops of rosehip oil.
2. Optionally, add a drop of ylang-ylang or lavender essential oil for a soothing aroma.
3. Close the bottle or container tightly and shake well to mix the ingredients.

Usage:

1. After cleansing your face, apply a small amount of the argan oil serum to your skin.
2. Gently massage the serum into your skin until fully absorbed.
3. Allow the serum to dry before applying moisturizer or other skincare products.

Storage:

- Store the argan oil serum in a small, dark-colored glass bottle with a dropper for easy application.
- Keep the bottle tightly sealed to protect the oils from oxidation.
- Store in a cool, dark place, away from direct sunlight and heat sources.

- Use within 6-12 months for optimal freshness and potency.

Note: Essential oils can cause skin irritation in some individuals. Perform a patch test before using, especially if you have sensitive skin or allergies. Discontinue use if any irritation occurs.

Ingredients:

- 1 tablespoon grapeseed oil
- A few drops of vitamin E oil
- Optional: a drop or two of chamomile or rose essential oil

Instructions:

1. In a small bottle or container, combine 1 tablespoon of grapeseed oil with a few drops of vitamin E oil.
2. Optionally, add a drop or two of chamomile or rose essential oil for a calming effect.
3. Close the bottle or container tightly and shake well to mix the ingredients.

Usage:

1. After cleansing your face, apply a small amount of the grapeseed oil serum to your skin.
2. Gently massage the serum into your skin until fully absorbed.
3. Allow the serum to dry before applying moisturizer or other skincare products.

Storage:

- Store the grapeseed oil serum in a small, dark-colored glass bottle with a dropper for easy application.
- Keep the bottle tightly sealed to protect the oils from oxidation.

- Store in a cool, dark place, away from direct sunlight and heat sources.
- Use within 6-12 months for optimal freshness and potency.

Note: Essential oils can cause skin irritation in some individuals. Perform a patch test before using, especially if you have sensitive skin or allergies. Discontinue use if any irritation occurs.

FACE MASKS AND SCRUBS

DIY face masks and scrubs provide a convenient and affordable way to care for your skin using natural ingredients. Face masks deeply cleanse and nourish the skin, while scrubs help exfoliate and renew its texture. Creating these products at home allows you to tailor them to your specific skin type and concerns, ensuring effective and personalized skincare.

There are various DIY face mask options available. Clay masks, such as bentonite or kaolin clay-based ones, are excellent for oily or acne-prone skin as they draw out impurities and excess oil. For dry or sensitive skin, masks with ingredients like honey, yogurt, or avocado can provide soothing and moisturizing benefits. Adding tea tree oil, turmeric, or aloe vera gel can address specific concerns like acne, inflammation or hyperpigmentation.

DIY scrubs are great for removing dead skin cells and improving skin texture. Common ingredients like sugar, salt, coffee grounds or ground oats serve as natural exfoliants. Mix them with carrier oils like coconut, olive, or almond oil, and add essential oils for additional benefits and a pleasant scent. Be gentle when using scrubs to avoid over-exfoliation, especially if you have sensitive skin.

Maintaining proper hygiene is crucial when preparing DIY face masks and scrubs. Ensure clean hands and tools, and use fresh ingredients to prevent contamination. Patch testing on a small area of your skin before application is recommended, especially for sensitive skin or known allergies. Also, be mindful of the storage and shelf life of your homemade products, as some ingredients may have a limited lifespan.

DIY face masks and scrubs offer an affordable and customizable approach to skincare. By using natural ingredients, you can care for your skin without exposure to harsh chemicals. However, remember that these homemade treatments should not replace professional skincare advice, especially for severe skin conditions. If you have concerns or persistent skin issues, consulting with a dermatologist or skincare professional is always recommended.

Ingredients:

- 1 tablespoon honey
- 1 tablespoon plain yogurt

Instructions:

1. In a small bowl, mix 1 tablespoon of honey with 1 tablespoon of plain yogurt.
2. Stir the ingredients until well combined and smooth.

Usage:

1. Cleanse your face before applying the mask.
2. Using clean fingers or a brush, apply the honey and yogurt mixture to your face.
3. Gently massage the mask into your skin in circular motions.
4. Leave the mask on for 15-20 minutes.
5. Rinse off the mask with lukewarm water and pat your face dry.

Storage:

- The mask is best used immediately after preparation.
- If there is any leftover mask, you can store it in an airtight container in the refrigerator for up to 2 days.
- Before using the stored mask, allow it to come to room temperature and give it a stir.

Note: Perform a patch test before using the mask, especially if you have allergies or sensitive skin. Discontinue use if any irritation occurs.

Ingredients:

- 1/2 ripe banana
- 1 tablespoon oatmeal
- 1 teaspoon honey

Instructions:

1. In a small bowl, mash half a ripe banana until it becomes a smooth paste.
2. Add 1 tablespoon of oatmeal and 1 teaspoon of honey to the mashed banana.
3. Stir the ingredients until well combined.

Usage:

1. Cleanse your face before applying the mask.
2. Using clean fingers or a brush, apply the oatmeal and banana mixture to your face.
3. Gently massage the mask into your skin in circular motions.
4. Leave the mask on for 15-20 minutes.
5. Rinse off the mask with lukewarm water and pat your face dry.

Storage:

- The mask is best used immediately after preparation.
- If there is any leftover mask, you can store it in an airtight container in the refrigerator for up to 2 days.

- Before using the stored mask, allow it to come to room temperature and give it a stir.

Note: Perform a patch test before using the mask, especially if you have allergies or sensitive skin. Discontinue use if any irritation occurs.

Ingredients:

- 1/2 ripe avocado
- 1 tablespoon honey

Instructions:

1. In a small bowl, scoop out the flesh of half a ripe avocado.
2. Mash the avocado with a fork until it becomes a smooth paste.
3. Add 1 tablespoon of honey to the mashed avocado.
4. Stir the ingredients until well combined.

Usage:

1. Cleanse your face before applying the mask.
2. Using clean fingers or a brush, apply the avocado and honey mixture to your face.
3. Gently massage the mask into your skin in circular motions.
4. Leave the mask on for 15-20 minutes.
5. Rinse off the mask with lukewarm water and pat your face dry.

Storage:

- The mask is best used immediately after preparation.
- If there is any leftover mask, you can store it in an airtight container in the refrigerator for up to 2 days.

- Before using the stored mask, allow it to come to room temperature and give it a stir.

Note: Perform a patch test before using the mask, especially if you have allergies or sensitive skin. Discontinue use if any irritation occurs.

Ingredients:

- 1 teaspoon turmeric powder
- 1 tablespoon plain yogurt

Instructions:

1. In a small bowl, combine 1 teaspoon of turmeric powder with 1 tablespoon of plain yogurt.
2. Stir the ingredients until well combined and smooth.

Usage:

1. Cleanse your face before applying the mask.
2. Using clean fingers or a brush, apply the turmeric and yogurt mixture to your face.
3. Gently massage the mask into your skin in circular motions.
4. Leave the mask on for 15-20 minutes.
5. Rinse off the mask with lukewarm water and pat your face dry.

Storage:

- The mask is best used immediately after preparation.
- If there is any leftover mask, you can store it in an airtight container in the refrigerator for up to 2 days.
- Before using the stored mask, allow it to come to room temperature and give it a stir.

Note: Turmeric can stain fabric and surfaces, so take care when using this mask. Perform a patch test before using the mask, especially if you have allergies or sensitive skin. Discontinue use if any irritation occurs.

Ingredients:

- 1/2 cucumber
- 2 tablespoons aloe vera gel

Instructions:

1. Peel and chop half a cucumber into small pieces.
2. Blend the cucumber pieces in a blender or food processor until smooth.
3. Transfer the blended cucumber to a small bowl.
4. Add 2 tablespoons of aloe vera gel to the bowl.
5. Stir the ingredients until well combined.

Usage:

1. Cleanse your face before applying the mask.
2. Using clean fingers or a brush, apply the cucumber and aloe vera mixture to your face.
3. Gently massage the mask into your skin in circular motions.
4. Leave the mask on for 15-20 minutes.
5. Rinse off the mask with lukewarm water and pat your face dry.

Storage:

- The mask is best used immediately after preparation.
- If there is any leftover mask, you can store it in an airtight container in the refrigerator for up to 2 days.

- Before using the stored mask, allow it to come to
  room temperature and give it a stir.

Note: Perform a patch test before using the mask, especially if you have allergies or sensitive skin. Discontinue
use if any irritation occurs.

Ingredients:

- 1/2 cup sugar
- 2 tablespoons olive oil
- Optional: a few drops of essential oil (such as lavender or peppermint) for fragrance

Instructions:

1. In a small bowl, combine 1/2 cup of sugar with 2 tablespoons of olive oil.
2. Optional: Add a few drops of essential oil for fragrance and mix well.

Usage:

1. Wet your skin in the shower or bath.
2. Take a small amount of the sugar and olive oil scrub and apply it to your body or face.
3. Gently massage the scrub into your skin using circular motions for a few minutes.
4. Rinse off the scrub with warm water.
5. Follow up with a moisturizer to nourish your skin.

Storage:

- Transfer any remaining scrub into an airtight container.
- Store the container in a cool, dry place away from direct sunlight.
- Use within 1-2 months for optimal freshness.

Note: Avoid using the scrub on broken or irritated skin. Perform a patch test before using the scrub, especially if

you have sensitive skin. Discontinue use if any irritation occurs.

Ingredients:
- 1/2 cup used coffee grounds
- 2 tablespoons melted coconut oil
- Optional: 1 teaspoon honey for added moisturization

Instructions:
1. In a small bowl, combine 1/2 cup of used coffee grounds with 2 tablespoons of melted coconut oil.
2. Optional: Add 1 teaspoon of honey to the mixture for added moisturization.
3. Mix the ingredients well until they are thoroughly combined.

Usage:
1. Wet your skin in the shower or bath.
2. Take a small amount of the coffee grounds and coconut oil scrub and apply it to your body or face.
3. Gently massage the scrub into your skin using circular motions for a few minutes.
4. Rinse off the scrub with warm water.
5. Follow up with a moisturizer to nourish your skin.

Storage:
- Transfer any remaining scrub into an airtight container.
- Store the container in a cool, dry place away from direct sunlight.

- Use within 1-2 months for optimal freshness.

Note: Avoid using the scrub on broken or irritated skin. Perform a patch test before using the scrub, especially if you have sensitive skin. Discontinue use if any irritation occurs.

Ingredients:

- 1/2 cup sea salt
- 2 tablespoons grapefruit juice
- Optional: 1 teaspoon olive oil for added moisture

Instructions:

1. In a small bowl, combine 1/2 cup of sea salt with 2 tablespoons of grapefruit juice.
2. Optional: Add 1 teaspoon of olive oil to the mixture for added moisture.
3. Stir the ingredients until well combined.

Usage:

1. Wet your skin in the shower or bath.
2. Take a small amount of the sea salt and grapefruit scrub and apply it to your body or face.
3. Gently massage the scrub into your skin using circular motions for a few minutes.
4. Rinse off the scrub with warm water.
5. Follow up with a moisturizer to nourish your skin.

Storage:

- Transfer any remaining scrub into an airtight container.
- Store the container in a cool, dry place away from direct sunlight.
- Use within 1-2 months for optimal freshness.

Note: Avoid using the scrub on broken or irritated skin. Perform a patch test before using the scrub, especially if

you have sensitive skin. Discontinue use if any irritation occurs.

Ingredients:

- 1/2 cup brown sugar
- 2 tablespoons honey
- Optional: a few drops of vanilla extract for scent

Instructions:

1. In a small bowl, combine 1/2 cup of brown sugar with 2 tablespoons of honey.
2. Optional: Add a few drops of vanilla extract for a pleasant scent and mix well.

Usage:

1. Wet your skin in the shower or bath.
2. Take a small amount of the brown sugar and honey scrub and apply it to your body or face.
3. Gently massage the scrub into your skin using circular motions for a few minutes.
4. Rinse off the scrub with warm water.
5. Follow up with a moisturizer to nourish your skin.

Storage:

- Transfer any remaining scrub into an airtight container.
- Store the container in a cool, dry place away from direct sunlight.
- Use within 1-2 months for optimal freshness.

Note: Avoid using the scrub on broken or irritated skin. Perform a patch test before using the scrub, especially if

you have sensitive skin. Discontinue use if any irritation occurs.

Ingredients:
- 1/2 cup almond meal
- 2 tablespoons plain yogurt
- Optional: 1 teaspoon lemon juice for brightening effect

Instructions:
1. In a small bowl, combine 1/2 cup of almond meal with 2 tablespoons of plain yogurt.
2. Optional: Add 1 teaspoon of lemon juice to the mixture for a brightening effect.
3. Mix the ingredients until well combined.

Usage:
1. Wet your skin in the shower or bath.
2. Take a small amount of the almond meal and yogurt scrub and apply it to your body or face.
3. Gently massage the scrub into your skin using circular motions for a few minutes.
4. Rinse off the scrub with warm water.
5. Follow up with a moisturizer to nourish your skin.

Storage:
- Transfer any remaining scrub into an airtight container.
- Store the container in a cool, dry place away from direct sunlight.
- Use within 1-2 months for optimal freshness.

Note: Avoid using the scrub on broken or irritated skin. Perform a patch test before using the scrub, especially if you have sensitive skin. Discontinue use if any irritation occurs.

LIP BALMS AND BODY BUTTERS

DIY lip balms and body butters are customizable skincare products that provide nourishment and hydration for your lips and body. Making these products at home allows you to use natural and gentle ingredients tailored to your preferences and needs.

For DIY lip balms, ingredients like beeswax, carrier oils (such as coconut or almond oil), and moisturizing elements like shea butter or cocoa butter are commonly used. These ingredients work together to create a smooth and hydrating balm that protects against dryness and chapping. You can also add natural flavors or essential oils for a pleasant scent.

Body butters are luxurious moisturizers that deeply nourish and soften the skin. They can be made with shea butter, cocoa butter, and carrier oils like coconut or jojoba oil. These ingredients provide essential fatty acids and vitamins for improved skin elasticity and moisture retention. Personalize your body butter by adding natural fragrances or essential oils.

Maintaining hygiene is important when making DIY lip balms and body butters. Use clean utensils and store the products in airtight containers to prevent contamination. Be mindful that homemade skincare products have a shorter shelf life, so monitor their freshness and discard any spoiled items.

DIY lip balms and body butters allow you to control the ingredients you apply to your skin. They offer effective hydration and protection without synthetic chemicals. However, always perform a patch test on a small area of skin, especially if you have sensitive skin or known allergies. Discontinue use if any adverse reactions occur.

These homemade products provide a cost-effective and sustainable option for lip and body care. Enjoy the process of exploring different ingredients and formulations to create personalized skincare products that nourish and pamper your lips and body.

Ingredients:

- 2 tablespoons coconut oil
- 1 tablespoon beeswax pellets
- Optional: a few drops of essential oil for fragrance (such as peppermint or lavender)

Instructions:

1. In a double boiler, melt 2 tablespoons of coconut oil and 1 tablespoon of beeswax pellets over low heat. Stir occasionally until completely melted and well combined.
2. Optional: Add a few drops of essential oil for fragrance and mix well.
3. Carefully pour the mixture into lip balm tubes or containers.
4. Allow the lip balm to cool and solidify at room temperature for a few hours.

Storage:

- Store the lip balm in a cool, dry place away from direct sunlight.
- It can last for several months if stored properly.
- To use, apply the lip balm to your lips as needed throughout the day.

Note: Be cautious when handling hot ingredients. Perform a patch test before applying the lip balm, especially if you have sensitive skin. Discontinue use if any irritation occurs.

Ingredients:

- 1 tablespoon shea butter
- 1 tablespoon almond oil
- Optional: a few drops of essential oil for fragrance (such as vanilla or citrus)

Instructions:

1. In a double boiler, melt 1 tablespoon of shea butter and 1 tablespoon of almond oil over low heat. Stir occasionally until completely melted and well combined.
2. Optional: Add a few drops of essential oil for fragrance and mix well.
3. Carefully pour the mixture into lip balm tubes or containers.
4. Allow the lip balm to cool and solidify at room temperature for a few hours.

Storage:

- Store the lip balm in a cool, dry place away from direct sunlight.
- It can last for several months if stored properly.
- To use, apply the lip balm to your lips as needed throughout the day.

Note: Be cautious when handling hot ingredients. Perform a patch test before applying the lip balm, especially if you have sensitive skin. Discontinue use if any irritation occurs.

Ingredients:
- 1 tablespoon honey
- 1 tablespoon olive oil
- Optional: a few drops of vitamin E oil for added nourishment

Instructions:
1. In a small bowl, mix 1 tablespoon of honey with 1 tablespoon of olive oil until well combined.
2. Optional: Add a few drops of vitamin E oil and stir well.
3. Carefully pour the mixture into lip balm tubes or containers.
4. Allow the lip balm to cool and solidify at room temperature for a few hours.

Storage:
- Store the lip balm in a cool, dry place away from direct sunlight.
- It can last for several months if stored properly.
- To use, apply the lip balm to your lips as needed throughout the day.

Note: Perform a patch test before applying the lip balm, especially if you have sensitive skin. Discontinue use if any irritation occurs.

Ingredients:

- 1 tablespoon cocoa butter
- 1 tablespoon coconut oil
- Optional: a few drops of vitamin E oil

Instructions:

1. In a double boiler, melt 1 tablespoon of cocoa butter and 1 tablespoon of coconut oil over low heat. Stir occasionally until completely melted and well combined.
2. Optional: Add a few drops of vitamin E oil and mix well.
3. Carefully pour the mixture into lip balm tubes or containers.
4. Allow the lip balm to cool and solidify at room temperature for a few hours.

Storage:

- Store the lip balm in a cool, dry place away from direct sunlight.
- It can last for several months if stored properly.
- To use, apply the lip balm to your lips as needed throughout the day.

Note: Be cautious when handling hot ingredients. Perform a patch test before applying the lip balm, especially if you have sensitive skin. Discontinue use if any irritation occurs.

Ingredients:

- 1/2 cup shea butter
- 1/4 cup coconut oil
- Optional: a few drops of essential oil for fragrance (such as lavender or vanilla)

Instructions:

1. In a double boiler, melt 1/2 cup of shea butter and 1/4 cup of coconut oil over low heat. Stir occasionally until completely melted and well combined.
2. Optional: Add a few drops of essential oil for fragrance and mix well.
3. Remove from heat and let the mixture cool to room temperature.
4. Transfer the cooled mixture to a mixing bowl and place it in the refrigerator for about 15-20 minutes, or until it starts to slightly solidify.
5. Using an electric mixer, whip the mixture on medium to high speed until it reaches a light and fluffy consistency.
6. Spoon the body butter into clean, airtight jars or containers.

Storage:

- Store the body butter in a cool, dry place away from direct sunlight.
- It can last for several months if stored properly.

- To use, apply a small amount to your skin and massage until absorbed.

Note: Perform a patch test before using the body butter, especially if you have sensitive skin. Discontinue use if any irritation occurs.

Ingredients:

- 1/2 cup cocoa butter
- 1/4 cup jojoba oil
- Optional: a few drops of essential oil for fragrance (such as lavender or peppermint)

Instructions:

1. In a double boiler, melt 1/2 cup of cocoa butter and 1/4 cup of jojoba oil over low heat. Stir occasionally until completely melted and well combined.
2. Optional: Add a few drops of essential oil for fragrance and mix well.
3. Remove from heat and let the mixture cool to room temperature.
4. Transfer the cooled mixture to a mixing bowl and place it in the refrigerator for about 15-20 minutes, or until it starts to slightly solidify.
5. Using an electric mixer, whip the mixture on medium to high speed until it reaches a light and fluffy consistency.
6. Spoon the body butter into clean, airtight jars or containers.

Storage:

- Store the body butter in a cool, dry place away from direct sunlight.
- It can last for several months if stored properly.

- To use, apply a small amount to your skin and massage until absorbed.

Note: Perform a patch test before using the body butter, especially if you have sensitive skin. Discontinue use if any irritation occurs.

Ingredients:

- 1/2 cup mango butter
- 1/4 cup sweet almond oil
- Optional: a few drops of essential oil for fragrance (such as citrus or jasmine)

Instructions:

1. In a double boiler, melt 1/2 cup of mango butter and 1/4 cup of sweet almond oil over low heat. Stir occasionally until completely melted and well combined.
2. Optional: Add a few drops of essential oil for fragrance and mix well.
3. Remove from heat and let the mixture cool to room temperature.
4. Transfer the cooled mixture to a mixing bowl and place it in the refrigerator for about 15-20 minutes, or until it starts to slightly solidify.
5. Using an electric mixer, whip the mixture on medium to high speed until it reaches a light and fluffy consistency.
6. Spoon the body butter into clean, airtight jars or containers.

Storage:

- Store the body butter in a cool, dry place away from direct sunlight.
- It can last for several months if stored properly.

- To use, apply a small amount to your skin and massage until absorbed.

Note: Perform a patch test before using the body butter, especially if you have sensitive skin. Discontinue use if any irritation occurs.

Ingredients:

- 1/2 cup avocado butter
- 1/4 cup argan oil
- Optional: a few drops of essential oil for fragrance (such as lavender or rose)

Instructions:

1. In a double boiler, melt 1/2 cup of avocado butter and 1/4 cup of argan oil over low heat. Stir occasionally until completely melted and well combined.
2. Optional: Add a few drops of essential oil for fragrance and mix well.
3. Remove from heat and let the mixture cool to room temperature.
4. Transfer the cooled mixture to a mixing bowl and place it in the refrigerator for about 15-20 minutes, or until it starts to slightly solidify.
5. Using an electric mixer, whip the mixture on medium to high speed until it reaches a light and fluffy consistency.
6. Spoon the body butter into clean, airtight jars or containers.

Storage:

- Store the body butter in a cool, dry place away from direct sunlight.
- It can last for several months if stored properly.

- To use, apply a small amount to your skin and massage until absorbed.

Note: Perform a patch test before using the body butter, especially if you have sensitive skin. Discontinue use if any irritation occurs.

Hair care products

DIY hair care products provide a natural and customizable approach to hair care. By creating your own products at home, you can avoid harsh chemicals and tailor the ingredients to meet your specific needs. From shampoos and conditioners to masks and treatments, DIY hair care is a cost-effective and sustainable way to nourish and enhance the health of your hair.

For homemade shampoos, ingredients like castile soap, aloe vera gel, and essential oils can be combined to create a gentle cleansing formula. Customizing the ingredients based on your hair type and concerns, such as dryness or oiliness, can help achieve optimal results.

DIY conditioners can be made using natural ingredients like coconut milk, shea butter and honey. These ingredients provide deep conditioning and moisturizing benefits, leaving your hair soft, smooth, and manageable. Adding ingredients like avocado, olive oil, or yogurt can further enhance nourishment and hydration.

Hair masks and treatments are popular DIY options. Ingredients such as coconut oil, argan oil, and honey can be used to create nourishing and repairing masks that address specific hair concerns like dryness, frizz or damage. Essential oils or herbal extracts can be incorporated for added benefits and fragrance.

It's important to understand your hair type and specific needs when experimenting with DIY hair care. Patch testing is crucial to identify potential allergies or sensitivities before applying homemade products to your scalp or hair.

While DIY hair care can be effective, it's advisable to seek professional guidance from a hair stylist or trichologist for severe hair concerns or conditions.

Embrace the creativity of DIY hair care as you discover the joy of naturally nourishing and maintaining your hair. Experiment with different recipes, explore new ingredients, and enjoy the journey towards healthier, more beautiful hair.

Ingredients:

- Coconut oil (enough to coat your hair)

Instructions:

1. Melt the coconut oil in a microwave-safe bowl or by placing the jar in warm water until it liquefies.
2. Part your hair into sections and apply the melted coconut oil to your scalp and hair, focusing on the ends.
3. Massage the oil into your scalp and work it through your hair using your fingers or a wide-toothed comb.
4. Once your hair is fully coated, cover it with a shower cap or towel to trap heat and enhance the conditioning effects.
5. Leave the hair mask on for at least 30 minutes, or overnight for an intense treatment.
6. After the desired time, shampoo your hair thoroughly to remove the oil. You may need to shampoo twice to ensure all the oil is removed.
7. Condition your hair as usual.

Storage:

- Store any leftover melted coconut oil in a sealed container at room temperature.
- It can last for a long time without refrigeration.

Note: Coconut oil tends to solidify in cooler temperatures. If the oil solidifies, warm it up before use by placing the

container in warm water or gently heating it in the micro-
wave.

Ingredients:

- 1 part apple cider vinegar
- 2 parts water

Instructions:

1. Mix 1 part apple cider vinegar with 2 parts water in a container or spray bottle.
2. After shampooing your hair, pour the apple cider vinegar rinse onto your hair and scalp.
3. Gently massage the mixture into your scalp for a few minutes.
4. Let the rinse sit in your hair for a couple of minutes.
5. Rinse your hair thoroughly with cool water to remove the vinegar smell.
6. Follow up with conditioner if desired.
7. Repeat once or twice a month or as needed.

Storage:

- Store the apple cider vinegar rinse in a sealed container at room temperature.
- It can last for a long time without refrigeration.

Note: If you have sensitive skin or a sensitive scalp, you may want to dilute the apple cider vinegar even further or perform a patch test before using it on your hair.

Ingredients:
- 1 ripe avocado
- 1 ripe banana

Instructions:
1. Mash the ripe avocado and banana together in a bowl until you achieve a smooth consistency.
2. Apply the mixture to your damp hair, starting from the roots and working your way to the ends.
3. Gently massage the mask into your scalp and hair, ensuring even coverage.
4. Once your hair is fully coated, cover it with a shower cap or towel to trap heat and enhance the conditioning effects.
5. Leave the hair mask on for 30 minutes to 1 hour.
6. Rinse your hair thoroughly with lukewarm water to remove the mask.
7. Shampoo and condition your hair as usual.

Storage:
- Use the mask immediately after preparing it for the best results.
- Discard any leftover mask, as it is best to make a fresh batch each time.

Note: You can adjust the ingredient measurements based on the length and thickness of your hair. Feel free to add a few drops of your favorite essential oil for a pleasant fragrance.

Ingredients:

- Aloe vera gel (from a fresh aloe vera leaf or store-bought)
- Optional: a few drops of your favorite essential oil for fragrance

Instructions:

1. Slice open a fresh aloe vera leaf and extract the gel using a spoon. Alternatively, use store-bought aloe vera gel.
2. If using fresh aloe vera gel, blend it in a blender or food processor until smooth. If using store-bought gel, skip this step.
3. Optional: Add a few drops of your favorite essential oil for fragrance and mix well.
4. Apply a small amount of the aloe vera gel to your hair, focusing on the areas that need hold or taming.
5. Style your hair as desired.
6. Allow the gel to air dry, or use a diffuser on low heat to speed up the drying process.

Storage:

- Store any unused aloe vera gel in an airtight container in the refrigerator.
- It can last for a few weeks if stored properly.

Note: Perform a patch test before applying the aloe vera gel to your hair, especially if you have sensitive skin or are allergic to aloe vera.

Ingredients:
- 2 tablespoons olive oil
- 1 tablespoon honey

Instructions:
1. In a small bowl, mix 2 tablespoons of olive oil with 1 tablespoon of honey until well combined.
2. Dampen your hair with water.
3. Apply the mixture to your hair, focusing on the ends and areas that need extra conditioning.
4. Gently massage the mixture into your hair and scalp.
5. Once your hair is fully coated, cover it with a shower cap or towel to trap heat and enhance the conditioning effects.
6. Leave the deep conditioning treatment on for 30 minutes to 1 hour.
7. Rinse your hair thoroughly with lukewarm water to remove the mixture.
8. Shampoo and condition your hair as usual.

Storage:
- Prepare the deep conditioning treatment immediately before use for the best results.
- Discard any leftover mixture, as it is best to make a fresh batch each time.

Note: Adjust the ingredient measurements based on your
hair length and thickness. Feel free to add a few drops of
your favorite essential oil for a pleasant fragrance.

CHAPTER 5: ADVANCED DIY SKINCARE RECIPES

ANTI-AGING TREATMENTS

DIY anti-aging treatments offer a natural and cost-effective way to address signs of aging and promote youthful-looking skin. By creating your own treatments at home, you can customize the ingredients to target specific concerns and nourish your skin with the power of natural ingredients.

One popular DIY anti-aging treatment is the use of serums. Serums are lightweight formulations that penetrate deeply into the skin, delivering potent ingredients that help reduce fine lines, wrinkles and promote a more youthful complexion. Ingredients like vitamin C, hyaluronic acid, and peptides are commonly used in DIY anti-aging serums to boost collagen production, improve elasticity and hydrate the skin.

Another DIY anti-aging treatment is the use of facial masks. Masks enriched with ingredients like retinol, green tea extract, or natural fruit enzymes can help exfoliate the skin, stimulate cell turnover, and promote a smoother and more radiant complexion. These masks provide intense nourishment and help diminish the appearance of fine lines and wrinkles.

Regular exfoliation is also crucial in anti-aging skincare. DIY scrubs made with gentle exfoliants like sugar, coffee grounds, or finely ground oatmeal can help remove dead skin cells, promote cell renewal, and improve the texture and tone of your skin. Exfoliating the skin regularly can reduce the appearance of fine lines and enhance the absorption of anti-aging ingredients.

When creating DIY anti-aging treatments, it's important to consider your skin's specific needs and sensitivities. Perform patch tests to ensure your skin doesn't react negatively to any ingredients. Additionally, be consistent with your skincare routine and maintain a healthy lifestyle with a balanced diet, regular exercise and adequate hydration for optimal results.

While DIY anti-aging treatments can provide effective results, it's important to note that they may not be as potent as professional treatments. For severe concerns or if you're unsure about specific ingredients, consult with a dermatologist or skincare professional for personalized advice.

Embrace the power of DIY anti-aging treatments as you care for your skin and combat signs of aging naturally. Enjoy the process of experimenting with different ingredients and formulations, and discover the joy of maintaining youthful and radiant skin in a sustainable and personalized way.

Ingredients:

- 1/4 teaspoon hyaluronic acid powder
- 2 tablespoons distilled water

Instructions:

1. In a small bottle or container, add 1/4 teaspoon of hyaluronic acid powder.
2. Gradually pour 2 tablespoons of distilled water into the container, stirring gently as you go.
3. Continue stirring until the hyaluronic acid powder is fully dissolved.
4. Let the serum sit for about 1 hour to allow the mixture to fully hydrate and thicken.
5. After an hour, give the serum a final stir to ensure it is well combined.
6. Apply a few drops of the serum to your face, focusing on areas where you want to target signs of aging.
7. Gently pat the serum into your skin and allow it to absorb.
8. Follow with your regular moisturizer or sunscreen.

Storage:

- Store the hyaluronic acid serum in a small, airtight bottle or container.
- Keep it in a cool, dark place away from direct sunlight or heat.

- The serum can last for approximately 1 to 2 weeks if stored properly.

Note: It's important to perform a patch test before using hyaluronic acid on your skin, especially if you have sensitive skin or are prone to allergies. Discontinue use if any irritation occurs.

Ingredients:

- 1 tablespoon glycolic acid
- 1 tablespoon distilled water
- 1 tablespoon aloe vera gel

Instructions:

1. In a small bowl, combine 1 tablespoon of glycolic acid, 1 tablespoon of distilled water, and 1 tablespoon of aloe vera gel.
2. Mix the ingredients thoroughly until they are well combined.
3. Cleanse your face and pat it dry.
4. Using a brush or cotton pad, apply a thin layer of the glycolic acid peel solution to your face, avoiding the eye area.
5. Leave the peel on for 5-10 minutes, or as directed on the glycolic acid product instructions.
6. Rinse your face thoroughly with cool water to neutralize the peel.
7. Follow with a gentle cleanser and moisturizer.
8. Apply sunscreen before going outside, as glycolic acid can increase skin sensitivity to the sun.

Storage:

- Store any unused portion of the glycolic acid peel solution in a sealed container in the refrigerator.
- It is best to make a fresh batch each time you want to use it.

- Discard any leftover solution after a single use.

Note: Glycolic acid is a potent ingredient and may cause irritation, especially for those with sensitive skin. It's essential to perform a patch test before using the peel and follow the instructions carefully. If any adverse reactions occur, discontinue use.

Ingredients:

- 1/2 teaspoon retinol powder
- 2 tablespoons aloe vera gel
- 1 tablespoon vitamin E oil

Instructions:

1. In a small bowl, combine 1/2 teaspoon of retinol powder, 2 tablespoons of aloe vera gel, and 1 tablespoon of vitamin E oil.
2. Mix the ingredients well until they are thoroughly combined.
3. Cleanse your face and pat it dry.
4. Apply a few drops of the retinol serum to your face, focusing on areas of concern.
5. Gently massage the serum into your skin using upward circular motions.
6. Allow the serum to absorb fully before applying any other skincare products.
7. Use the retinol serum in the evening, as it may increase sun sensitivity.
8. Follow with a moisturizer if needed.

Storage:

- Store the retinol face serum in a dark, airtight container.
- Keep it in a cool, dry place away from direct sunlight.

- The serum can last for approximately 2 to 3 weeks if stored properly.

Note: Retinol is a powerful ingredient and may cause skin sensitivity or irritation, especially for those with sensitive skin. Start with a lower concentration and gradually increase usage as tolerated. Always perform a patch test before applying the serum to your face.

Ingredients:

- 1 tablespoon plain Greek yogurt
- 1 tablespoon honey
- 1 teaspoon lemon juice
- 1 teaspoon rosehip oil

Instructions:

1. In a small bowl, combine 1 tablespoon of plain Greek yogurt, 1 tablespoon of honey, 1 teaspoon of lemon juice, and 1 teaspoon of rosehip oil.
2. Mix the ingredients well until they form a smooth paste.
3. Cleanse your face and pat it dry.
4. Apply a thick layer of the collagen-boosting mask to your face, avoiding the eye area.
5. Leave the mask on for 15-20 minutes.
6. Rinse off the mask with warm water, gently massaging your skin in circular motions.
7. Follow with your regular skincare routine, including moisturizer.
8. Use the mask 1-2 times a week for best results.

Storage:

- Use the collagen-boosting mask immediately after preparing it for the best results.
- Discard any leftover mask, as it is best to make a fresh batch each time.

Note: Perform a patch test before using the mask, especially if you have sensitive skin or are allergic to any of the ingredients. Discontinue use if any irritation occurs.

Ingredients:

- 1 tablespoon rosehip oil
- 1 tablespoon argan oil
- 1 tablespoon jojoba oil
- 5 drops lavender essential oil
- 3 drops geranium essential oil

Instructions:

1. In a small glass bottle or container, combine 1 tablespoon of rosehip oil, 1 tablespoon of argan oil, and 1 tablespoon of jojoba oil.
2. Add 5 drops of lavender essential oil and 3 drops of geranium essential oil to the mixture.
3. Secure the bottle with a lid and shake well to ensure all the oils are thoroughly mixed.
4. Cleanse your face and pat it dry.
5. Apply a few drops of the hydrating facial oil to your fingertips.
6. Gently massage the oil onto your face, focusing on dry or aging areas.
7. Allow the oil to absorb into your skin for a few minutes before applying other skincare products.
8. Use the facial oil in the evening or as needed for intense hydration.

Storage:

- Store the hydrating facial oil in a cool, dark place away from direct sunlight.

- Ensure the bottle or container is tightly sealed to prevent air and light exposure.
- The oil can last for approximately 6 months if stored properly.

Note: Perform a patch test before using the facial oil, especially if you have sensitive skin or are prone to allergies. Discontinue use if any irritation occurs.

ACNE-FIGHTING SOLUTIONS

DIY acne-fighting solutions offer a natural and customizable approach to tackling acne and promoting clearer skin. These homemade remedies provide the opportunity to address acne concerns using readily available ingredients without relying on commercial products that may contain harsh chemicals.

One popular DIY option is spot treatments, which are targeted solutions designed to reduce the size and redness of individual acne lesions. Ingredients like tea tree oil, witch hazel, and aloe vera gel possess antibacterial and anti-inflammatory properties that can help combat acne-causing bacteria and soothe irritated skin.

Another effective DIY option is acne-fighting masks, which can be formulated using ingredients such as clay, activated charcoal, and honey. These ingredients work together to draw out impurities, absorb excess oil, and calm inflammation, resulting in a clearer complexion.

Additionally, DIY cleansers can be customized to address acne-prone skin. Ingredients like salicylic acid, neem oil, and grapefruit extract help exfoliate dead skin cells, control oil production, and unclog pores, reducing the occurrence of breakouts.

It's important to note that while DIY acne-fighting solutions can be beneficial for mild to moderate acne, severe or persistent acne may require professional guidance. Consulting with a dermatologist can provide personalized advice and treatment options tailored to your specific skin condition.

Incorporating DIY acne-fighting solutions into your skincare routine allows you to take an active role in caring for your skin and promoting a clearer complexion naturally. By experimenting with different ingredients and formulations, you can find the most effective solution for your skin's unique needs. With consistency and patience, DIY acne-fighting solutions can help you achieve healthier, blemish-free skin.

Ingredients:

- 2 tablespoons salicylic acid solution (2% concentration)
- 4 tablespoons distilled water
- 1 tablespoon aloe vera gel

Instructions:

1. In a small bowl, mix 2 tablespoons of salicylic acid solution with 4 tablespoons of distilled water.
2. Add 1 tablespoon of aloe vera gel to the mixture and stir well to combine.
3. Cleanse your face and pat it dry.
4. Using a brush or cotton pad, apply a thin layer of the salicylic acid peel solution to your face, avoiding the eye area.
5. Leave the peel on for the recommended time as per the salicylic acid product instructions. Start with a shorter time for your first peel to assess tolerance.
6. Rinse your face thoroughly with cool water to neutralize the peel.
7. Apply a soothing moisturizer or aloe vera gel to calm the skin.
8. Use the salicylic acid peel once a week or as directed, gradually increasing the duration and frequency based on your skin's response.

Storage:

- Store the salicylic acid peel solution in a dark, air-tight container.
- Keep it in a cool, dry place away from direct sunlight.
- Discard any unused solution after a few weeks or as per the product expiration date.

Note: Salicylic acid peels are potent treatments and may cause skin sensitivity, redness, or peeling. It's crucial to perform a patch test before using the peel and follow the instructions carefully. If any adverse reactions occur, discontinue use.

Ingredients:

- 1 tablespoon bentonite clay
- 1 tablespoon apple cider vinegar
- 1-2 drops tea tree essential oil (optional)
- Water (as needed)

Instructions:

1. In a non-metallic bowl, mix 1 tablespoon of bentonite clay with 1 tablespoon of apple cider vinegar.
2. Add 1-2 drops of tea tree essential oil (optional) for its antibacterial properties.
3. Gradually add water to the mixture, stirring well until you achieve a smooth paste-like consistency.
4. Cleanse your face and pat it dry.
5. Apply a thick, even layer of the bentonite clay mask to your face, avoiding the eye and lip areas.
6. Allow the mask to dry for 10-15 minutes or until it starts to feel tight on your skin.
7. Rinse your face with warm water to remove the mask, gently massaging in circular motions.
8. Pat your skin dry and follow with a light moisturizer.

Storage:

- As bentonite clay masks are best used when freshly mixed, it is recommended to prepare a new batch each time.

- Store any leftover clay powder in a sealed container in a cool, dry place away from moisture.

Note: Bentonite clay masks may cause temporary redness or slight tingling due to increased blood circulation. If you have sensitive skin, start with a patch test and consider reducing the frequency of use.

Garlic and Yogurt Spot Treatment

Ingredients:
- 1 clove of garlic
- 1 tablespoon plain yogurt

Instructions:
1. Peel and finely mince 1 clove of garlic.
2. In a small bowl, combine the minced garlic with 1 tablespoon of plain yogurt.
3. Mix well until the ingredients are thoroughly blended.
4. Cleanse your face and pat it dry.
5. Apply a small amount of the garlic and yogurt mixture directly to acne spots using a cotton swab or your fingertips.
6. Leave the spot treatment on for 10-15 minutes.
7. Rinse your face with cool water to remove the treatment.
8. Apply a soothing moisturizer to the treated areas.

Storage:
- Since this spot treatment is prepared fresh, it is recommended to use it immediately.
- Discard any leftover mixture, as it is best to make a fresh batch each time.

Note: Garlic may cause a tingling or stinging sensation on the skin. If you experience any discomfort or irritation, rinse off the treatment immediately. Perform a patch test before using the spot treatment, especially if you have sensitive or allergic skin.

Ingredients:
- 2-3 drops of neem oil
- 1 tablespoon of pure aloe vera gel

Instructions:
1. In a small bowl, mix 2-3 drops of neem oil with 1 tablespoon of pure aloe vera gel.
2. Stir well to ensure the ingredients are thoroughly combined.
3. Cleanse your face and pat it dry.
4. Apply a small amount of the neem oil and aloe vera gel mixture directly to acne spots using a cotton swab or your fingertips.
5. Gently massage the treatment into the affected areas.
6. Leave the spot treatment on for 15-20 minutes.
7. Rinse your face with cool water to remove the treatment.
8. Follow with your regular skincare routine.

Storage:
- Store the neem oil and aloe vera gel spot treatment in a cool, dark place away from direct sunlight.
- Ensure the container is tightly sealed to prevent air exposure.
- The mixture can be stored for up to 1 week in the refrigerator.

Note: Neem oil has a strong odor that may be unpleasant to some individuals. Perform a patch test before using the spot treatment, especially if you have sensitive or allergic skin. Discontinue use if any irritation or adverse reactions occur.

Tea Tree Oil Spot Treatment

Ingredients:
- Tea tree essential oil
- Carrier oil (such as jojoba oil or coconut oil)

Instructions:
1. In a small, clean container, mix 1-2 drops of tea tree essential oil with a carrier oil.
2. The ratio of tea tree oil to carrier oil should be around 1 drop of tea tree oil per 1 teaspoon of carrier oil.
3. Stir well to ensure the oils are blended.
4. Cleanse your face and pat it dry.
5. Using a cotton swab, apply a small amount of the spot treatment directly to acne spots.
6. Leave the treatment on overnight or for a few hours.
7. Rinse your face with cool water in the morning or after the recommended time.
8. Apply a light moisturizer to the treated areas.

Storage:
- Store the tea tree oil spot treatment in a cool, dry place away from direct sunlight.
- Ensure the container is tightly sealed to prevent air exposure.
- The mixture can be stored for several weeks.

Note: Tea tree oil is potent, so it's important to use it sparingly and always dilute it with a carrier oil. Perform a patch test before using the spot treatment, especially if you have sensitive or allergic skin. Discontinue use if any irritation or adverse reactions occur.

Natural remedies for specific skin conditions

Natural remedies offer a gentle and effective way to address specific skin conditions using readily available ingredients. These remedies harness the power of natural ingredients to provide relief and promote healthier skin.

For dry and dull skin, a moisturizing face mask using honey and avocado can provide deep hydration. Mix mashed avocado with honey, apply the mixture to your face, and leave it on for 15-20 minutes before rinsing. This mask helps nourish and replenish dry skin, leaving it soft and radiant.

To soothe irritated or sensitive skin, a chamomile and oatmeal face mask can provide relief. Brew chamomile tea and let it cool, then mix it with ground oatmeal to create a paste. Apply the mask to your face, leave it on for 10-15 minutes, and rinse gently. This mask helps calm inflammation and hydrate the skin.

For hyperpigmentation or dark spots, a lemon juice and honey brightening treatment can help lighten the skin. Mix fresh lemon juice with honey, apply it to the affected areas, and leave it on for 10-15 minutes before rinsing. Lemon juice acts as a natural bleaching agent, while honey helps moisturize the skin.

When dealing with oily skin, a clay mask using bentonite or kaolin clay can help absorb excess oil. Mix the clay with water or apple cider vinegar to form a paste, apply it to your face, and let it dry before rinsing. This mask helps remove impurities and control oil production.

It's important to note that natural remedies may not work for everyone, and individual results may vary. It's always recommended to perform a patch test before using any new ingredient on your skin, especially if you have sensitive or reactive skin. Additionally, if you have severe or persistent skin conditions, it's best to consult a dermatologist for personalized advice and treatment options.

Tea Tree Oil Spot Treatment for acne-prone skin:

Ingredients: Tea tree essential oil, carrier oil.

Instructions: Mix a few drops of tea tree oil with a carrier oil, apply to acne spots, and leave overnight.

Honey and Avocado Moisturizing Face Mask for dry and dull skin:

Ingredients: Avocado, honey.

Instructions: Mash avocado, mix with honey, apply to face, leave for 15-20 minutes, and rinse.

Chamomile and Oatmeal Soothing Face Mask for irritated or sensitive skin:

Ingredients: Chamomile tea, ground oatmeal.

Instructions: Brew chamomile tea, mix with oatmeal to form a paste, apply, leave for 10-15 minutes, and rinse.

Lemon Juice and Honey Brightening Treatment for hyperpigmentation:

Ingredients: Lemon juice, honey.

Instructions: Mix lemon juice with honey, apply to affected areas, leave for 10-15 minutes, and rinse.

Bentonite or Kaolin Clay Mask for oily skin:

Ingredients: Bentonite or kaolin clay, water or apple cider vinegar.

Instructions: Mix clay with water or vinegar, apply to face, let dry, and rinse.

Ingredients: Cucumber juice, mint leaves, distilled water.

Instructions: Blend cucumber and mint leaves, mix with water, and apply as a toner using a cotton pad.

Ingredients: Aloe vera gel, coconut oil.

Instructions: Mix aloe vera gel with coconut oil, apply to sunburned areas, and leave for relief.

Ingredients: Green tea leaves, rice water, castile soap (optional).

Instructions: Steep green tea, mix with rice water, and use as a facial cleanser.

Ingredients: Turmeric powder, yogurt, honey (optional).

Instructions: Mix turmeric, yogurt, and honey to form a paste, gently scrub onto the face, and rinse.

Ingredients: Rosewater, witch hazel, aloe vera gel (optional).

Instructions: Mix rosewater and witch hazel, add aloe vera gel (if desired), and use as a toning mist.

Sunscreen and natural SPF options

DIY homemade sunscreens and natural SPF options provide an alternative to commercially available products and allow you to customize the ingredients according to your preferences. While these options can provide some level of sun protection, it's important to note that they may not offer the same level of protection as commercially formulated sunscreens. Here are some elaborations on DIY homemade sunscreens and natural SPF options:

Zinc Oxide Sunscreen: Zinc oxide is a common ingredient in physical sunscreens as it provides broad-spectrum protection against both UVA and UVB rays. To make a zinc oxide sunscreen, mix zinc oxide powder with a carrier oil like coconut oil or shea butter. The ratio of zinc oxide to carrier oil will depend on the desired SPF level, but a typical starting point is 20% zinc oxide to 80% carrier oil. Store the sunscreen in a dark, airtight container. Remember to reapply it every two hours and after swimming or sweating.

Red Raspberry Seed Oil: Red raspberry seed oil has natural SPF properties and is rich in antioxidants. It offers some protection against UVA and UVB rays. However, it's important to note that the exact SPF level may vary, and additional sun protection measures should still be taken. Apply a small amount of red raspberry seed oil directly to the skin before sun exposure and reapply as needed.

Carrot Seed Oil: Carrot seed oil contains natural antioxidants and has a mild SPF value. It can be mixed with a carrier oil like jojoba or almond oil and applied to the skin for sun protection. However, it should be used in conjunction with other sun protection measures, as its SPF value may vary.

DIY Sunscreen Bars: You can also make sunscreen bars by combining ingredients like shea butter, coconut oil, beeswax, and a natural SPF booster like red raspberry seed oil or zinc oxide. Melt the ingredients together, pour the mixture into molds, and let it solidify. These bars provide a convenient way to apply sunscreen, especially for outdoor activities.

Additional Sun Protection Measures: Remember that DIY sunscreens and natural SPF options should not be the sole method of sun protection. It's important to take additional measures such as seeking shade during peak sun hours, wearing protective clothing, including hats and sunglasses, and using sun-protective umbrellas.

It's crucial to note that the effectiveness of DIY sunscreens and natural SPF options can vary, and they may not offer the same level of protection as commercially available sunscreens. If you have specific skin concerns or are spending extended time in the sun, it's advisable to consult a dermatologist or healthcare professional for personalized advice and guidance.

CHAPTER 6: CUSTOMIZING AND ADAPTING RECIPES

Understanding skin types and specific needs

Our skin is the largest organ of our body, and it plays a crucial role in protecting us from external factors such as environmental pollutants, harmful UV rays, and microbial infections. To maintain healthy and radiant skin, it is important to understand our individual skin type and cater to its specific needs. This knowledge allows us to develop a targeted skincare routine that addresses our skin's unique characteristics.

There are several common skin types: normal, dry, oily, combination, sensitive, and mature. Each skin type has distinct characteristics and requires different approaches to maintain its health and appearance.

Normal skin is well-balanced, with a smooth texture, small pores, and an even complexion. It requires regular cleansing to remove impurities, moisturizing to maintain hydration, and sun protection to prevent damage from harmful UV rays.

Dry skin lacks moisture and often feels tight, rough, or flaky. It requires gentle cleansers that do not strip away natural oils, as well as rich and emollient moisturizers to replenish lost moisture. Exfoliating regularly helps to remove dead skin cells and promote cell turnover.

Oily skin tends to produce excess sebum, resulting in a shiny appearance and a tendency for acne or breakouts. It benefits from cleansers that control oil production without over-drying the skin. Lightweight, oil-free moisturizers and products containing ingredients like salicylic acid or tea tree oil can help manage oiliness and prevent breakouts.

Combination skin is characterized by a mix of oily and dry areas. The T-zone (forehead, nose, and chin) tends to be oilier, while the cheeks are drier. Balancing cleansers and targeted products for each area, such as oil-controlling products for the T-zone and hydrating products for the cheeks, are beneficial.

Sensitive skin is easily irritated, prone to redness, and reacts to certain ingredients or environmental factors. It requires gentle and fragrance-free cleansers and moisturizers. Soothing ingredients like aloe vera or chamomile help to calm and protect sensitive skin. Patch testing new products is essential to prevent adverse reactions.

Mature skin experiences natural changes over time, including reduced elasticity, wrinkles, and age spots. It benefits from hydrating and nourishing products. Creamy cleansers and rich moisturizers help combat dryness, while ingredients like retinol, peptides, and antioxidants target signs of aging. Regular use of broad-spectrum sunscreen is crucial to protect mature skin from further damage.

In addition to understanding skin types, it is important to consider external factors such as climate, lifestyle, and hormonal changes, as they can affect the condition of our skin. Adjusting our skincare routine accordingly ensures that our skin receives the care it needs.

To effectively understand and address our skin's specific needs, it is beneficial to consult with a dermatologist or skincare professional who can provide personalized guidance. They can offer recommendations on suitable products, ingredients, and treatments based on our skin type, concerns and goals.

Understanding our skin type and its specific needs is the foundation of a healthy and effective skincare routine. By tailoring our skincare approach to our individual skin type, we can provide the necessary nourishment, hydration, and protection to achieve and maintain radiant and beautiful skin throughout our lives.

Modifying recipes for different skin concerns

When it comes to skincare, one size does not fit all. Each of us has unique skin concerns and conditions that require targeted care. Luckily, with the abundance of do-it-yourself (DIY) skincare recipes available, we can modify these recipes to address our specific skin concerns. By understanding the ingredients and their benefits, we can tailor our homemade skincare products to effectively target issues such as acne, dryness, hyperpigmentation and sensitivity.

Acne is a common concern for many individuals. To modify recipes for acne-prone skin, ingredients with anti-bacterial and anti-inflammatory properties can be incorporated. Tea tree oil, witch hazel, and salicylic acid are known for their ability to combat acne-causing bacteria and reduce inflammation. Consider adding a few drops of tea tree oil to cleansers or toners or including witch hazel as a toning ingredient in DIY recipes. For exfoliation, opt for gentle exfoliants like sugar or oatmeal, which help unclog pores without causing irritation.

Dry skin requires ingredients that provide deep hydration and nourishment. Modify recipes by including moisturizing ingredients such as shea butter, coconut oil, or hyaluronic acid. These ingredients help to replenish moisture, soothe dry patches, and restore the skin's natural barrier. Consider incorporating them into homemade moisturizers, serums, or masks. For added hydration, aloe vera gel or honey can be included as well.

Hyperpigmentation and uneven skin tone can be addressed by incorporating ingredients known for their brightening and clarifying properties. Lemon juice, vitamin C, and licorice extract are popular choices. These ingredients can be added to serums or masks to help fade dark spots and promote a more even complexion. However, it's important to use them in moderation and perform patch tests, as they can be sensitizing for some individuals.

Sensitive skin requires extra care and gentler ingredients. Modify recipes by choosing mild and soothing ingredients such as chamomile, cucumber, or oatmeal. These ingredients have calming properties and can help reduce redness and inflammation. Additionally, avoid using fragrances or harsh exfoliants that can irritate sensitive skin.

Modifying recipes for different skin concerns also involves adjusting the proportions of ingredients. For instance, if you have oily skin, you may want to reduce the amount of oil used in a moisturizer or choose lighter carrier oils like jojoba or grapeseed oil. On the other hand, if you have dry skin, you may increase the concentration of moisturizing ingredients or add a few drops of facial oil to your moisturizer.

Always remember to patch test any new ingredients or modified recipes to ensure you don't have any adverse reactions. Additionally, consult with a dermatologist or skincare professional if you have specific concerns or conditions that require professional guidance.

Modifying DIY skincare recipes for different skin concerns allows us to personalize our skincare routine and effectively address our unique needs. By incorporating ingredients that target specific concerns, adjusting proportions, and being mindful of potential sensitivities, we can create homemade products that provide the desired results. Understanding the benefits of different ingredients and experimenting with modifications empowers us to take control of our skincare journey and achieve healthier, more radiant skin.

Creating personalized skincare routines

Our skin is unique, and its needs can vary greatly from person to person. That's why creating a personalized skincare routine is essential to ensure that we are providing our skin with the care it deserves. By understanding our skin type, concerns, and goals, we can tailor our routine to address specific issues, promote healthy skin and achieve our desired results.

The first step in creating a personalized skincare routine is to determine our skin type. This helps us choose products and ingredients that are suitable for our specific needs. Common skin types include normal, dry, oily, combination, sensitive, and mature. Each type requires different approaches to achieve optimal health and balance.

Once we have identified our skin type, we can assess our skin concerns. These may include acne, dryness, oiliness, hyperpigmentation, sensitivity or signs of aging. Understanding our concerns allows us to select targeted products and treatments to address them effectively.

Building a personalized skincare routine involves a few key steps:

Cleansing: Choose a gentle cleanser that suits your skin type. Avoid harsh ingredients that can strip the skin of its natural oils. Cleansing should be done twice daily to remove impurities, excess oil and makeup.

Exfoliation: Incorporate exfoliation into your routine to remove dead skin cells and promote cell turnover. Choose an exfoliant that suits your skin type and concerns. Be mindful not to over-exfoliate, as it can cause irritation or dryness.

Toning: Use a toner to balance the skin's pH levels, remove any remaining impurities, and prepare the skin for further treatment. Look for toners that are alcohol-free and contain beneficial ingredients for your specific concerns.

Treatment: This step addresses specific skin concerns. It may involve serums, masks, or spot treatments. Choose products that target your concerns, whether it's acne, hydration, brightening, or anti-aging. Apply treatments according to the product instructions.

Moisturizing: Hydration is crucial for all skin types. Select a moisturizer that suits your skin type and provides the necessary hydration and nourishment. For daytime, choose a moisturizer with SPF to protect against harmful UV rays.

Sun Protection: Regardless of skin type or concerns, sun protection is vital. Use a broad-spectrum sunscreen with an appropriate SPF for your skin type. Apply it daily and reapply as needed, especially when spending time outdoors.

Eye Care: Incorporate an eye cream or serum to address specific concerns around the delicate eye area, such as fine lines, dark circles, or puffiness. Apply it gently using your ring finger.

Nighttime Routine: Before bedtime, follow the steps above, but with some modifications. Double cleanse to remove makeup and dirt thoroughly. Use a nighttime moisturizer or incorporate a specialized treatment, such as a retinol product, to address specific concerns while you sleep.

It's important to note that creating a personalized skincare routine is an ongoing process. Our skin changes with age, seasons, and other factors, so it's essential to reassess our routine periodically and make adjustments as needed.

Additionally, remember that consistency is key. Give your skincare routine time to work and be patient. Results may take time, so don't give up too quickly. Also, be cautious when introducing new products or ingredients, performing patch tests, and gradually incorporating them into your routine.

Seek advice from skincare professionals or dermatologists if you have specific concerns or conditions that require expert guidance. They can provide personalized recommendations and help you fine-tune your routine.

Creating a personalized skincare routine allows us to address our unique skin type, concerns, and goals. By selecting appropriate products, incorporating targeted treatments, and following a consistent regimen, we can nurture our skin's health and achieve the desired results. Remember, skincare is not one-size-fits-all, so take the time to understand your skin and develop a routine that works best for you.

CHAPTER 7: TROUBLESHOOT-ING AND COMMON FAQS

Addressing common issues in DIY skincare

DIY skincare has gained popularity as individuals seek natural and personalized solutions for their skincare needs. While DIY recipes offer numerous benefits, they can also present common issues that need to be addressed to ensure effective and safe skincare practices. By understanding and addressing these issues, we can maximize the benefits of DIY skincare and avoid potential pitfalls.

One common issue in DIY skincare is the lack of precision in ingredient measurements. Accurate measurements are crucial for the efficacy and safety of the final product. To address this issue, it is important to use precise measuring tools such as scales, measuring spoons, and droppers. Following the recipe instructions and adhering to the recommended ratios of ingredients will help ensure consistent and reliable results.

Another issue is the improper preservation of DIY skincare products. Without proper preservation, homemade products can become a breeding ground for bacteria, leading to contamination and potential skin irritations or infections. To address this, it is important to include effective natural preservatives in DIY skincare formulations, such as vitamin E oil, grapefruit seed extract, or essential oils with antimicrobial properties. Additionally, store the products in airtight containers and keep them in a cool, dry place to extend their shelf life.

Skin sensitivity and allergic reactions are also common issues in DIY skincare. Ingredients that are generally considered safe and beneficial for most individuals can still cause adverse reactions in some. To address this, perform patch tests before applying DIY products to the entire face or body. Apply a small amount of the product on a small patch of skin and observe for any adverse reactions or irritations. If a negative reaction occurs, discontinue use and consult with a dermatologist or healthcare professional.

Ensuring the quality and sourcing of ingredients is another important consideration in DIY skincare. Using high-quality, organic, and non-comedogenic ingredients can enhance the effectiveness and safety of the products. Research reputable suppliers and opt for ingredients that are free from pesticides, additives, and synthetic fragrances. Additionally, be mindful of expiration dates and storage recommendations for each ingredient to maintain their potency and effectiveness.

Proper documentation and record-keeping are essential in DIY skincare. Keep track of the ingredients used, their quantities, and any modifications made to the original recipes. This information can help identify any sensitivities or allergies, and allow for adjustments or improvements in future formulations.

Educating oneself on skincare science and understanding the specific needs of individual skin types and concerns is key to addressing common issues in DIY skincare. By learning about the properties and benefits of different ingredients, as well as their interactions with the skin, individuals can make informed decisions and modify recipes to suit their unique needs.

While DIY skincare offers numerous benefits, it is important to address common issues to ensure effective and safe practices. Precise ingredient measurements, proper preservation, consideration of skin sensitivity, sourcing high-quality ingredients, documentation, and education are all crucial elements to address these issues.

By addressing these concerns, individuals can enjoy the benefits of DIY skincare while minimizing potential risks and achieving healthier, more radiant skin naturally.

Troubleshooting ingredient interactions

In the world of DIY skincare, ingredient interactions play a significant role in the effectiveness and safety of home-made products. Understanding how different ingredients interact with one another is crucial to avoid potential issues and ensure desirable outcomes. However, occasionally, unexpected reactions or undesirable results may occur due to ingredient interactions. This is where troubleshooting becomes essential.

One common issue in DIY skincare is ingredient incompatibility. Certain ingredients may react adversely when combined, leading to instability, changes in texture or color, or even skin irritations. For instance, combining acidic ingredients like lemon juice with alkaline ingredients such as baking soda can result in a neutralization reaction, reducing the efficacy of both ingredients. To troubleshoot ingredient incompatibility, it is important to research and understand the pH levels of the ingredients being used. Avoid combining ingredients with vastly different pH levels, or consider using them in separate steps of your skincare routine to avoid interaction.

Another issue is ingredient sensitivity. Some individuals may experience adverse reactions or allergies to specific ingredients, even if they are generally considered safe. This can manifest as redness, irritation, or itching. To troubleshoot ingredient sensitivity, it is crucial to perform patch tests before applying the product to the entire face or body. Apply a small amount of the product to a small patch of skin, such as the inner forearm, and observe for any adverse reactions for at least 24 hours. If a negative reaction occurs, discontinue use and consult with a dermatologist or healthcare professional.

Texture and stability issues can also arise when certain ingredients are combined. For example, oil-based ingredients may separate from water-based ingredients, resulting in an unstable or unappealing product. To troubleshoot texture and stability issues, consider using emulsifiers or stabilizers that can help bind the ingredients together. Be sure to follow proper mixing techniques and ratios specified in the recipe.

It is important to note that some ingredients may enhance or diminish the efficacy of others. For instance, antioxidants like vitamin C can enhance the effectiveness of sunscreen ingredients, while certain essential oils may increase the skin's sensitivity to the sun. To troubleshoot such issues, it is crucial to research the properties and interactions of each ingredient being used. Adjust the concentrations or application methods accordingly to achieve the desired results.

When troubleshooting ingredient interactions, documentation is essential. Keep track of the ingredients used in each recipe, their ratios, and any modifications made. This allows for easier identification of potential problematic combinations and helps refine future formulations.

When troubleshooting ingredient interactions, it is essential to rely on reputable sources of information. Consult reliable skincare resources, scientific studies, and trusted experts to gain a better understanding of ingredient interactions and their potential effects on the skin.

Troubleshooting ingredient interactions is crucial in DIY skincare to achieve desirable outcomes and ensure the safety and effectiveness of homemade products. By understanding ingredient compatibility, conducting patch tests, addressing texture and stability issues, considering ingredient efficacy, and documenting the process, individuals can troubleshoot and refine their formulations. With proper knowledge and attention to detail, DIY skincare enthusiasts can create effective and customized products that cater to their specific skincare needs while minimizing potential risks.

As DIY skincare continues to gain popularity, individuals have many questions regarding its benefits, safety, and effectiveness. Addressing these frequently asked questions can help individuals make informed decisions and navigate the world of DIY skincare with confidence. Let's explore some common questions and provide detailed answers to them.

Is DIY skincare safe?

DIY skincare can be safe when proper precautions are taken. It is essential to research ingredients, follow reliable recipes, and practice good hygiene. Patch testing is also recommended to check for any adverse reactions or sensitivities before applying products to the entire face or body.

What are the benefits of DIY skincare?

DIY skincare offers several benefits. It allows individuals to customize products according to their specific needs, control the ingredients used, and avoid potential harmful additives or irritants found in commercial products. DIY skincare can also be cost-effective and environmentally friendly.

Can DIY skincare be as effective as commercial products?

DIY skincare can be effective when formulated with the right ingredients and in appropriate concentrations. However, it's important to manage expectations as the results may vary depending on individual factors such as skin type, specific concerns, and consistency of use.

How do I choose the right ingredients for my DIY skincare?

Choosing the right ingredients for DIY skincare involves considering your skin type, specific concerns, and the desired effects. Researching the properties and benefits of different ingredients can help in selecting the ones that target your specific needs.

Can I mix different DIY skincare recipes together?

It is generally recommended to follow recipes as they are formulated to provide specific results. Mixing different recipes together may alter the proportions and effectiveness of the ingredients. However, some ingredients can be combined safely, while others may interact negatively. Researching the compatibility of ingredients and performing small-scale experiments is advisable.

How can I address allergies or sensitivities in DIY skincare?

Individuals with allergies or sensitivities should be cautious when using new ingredients. Patch testing is crucial to identify potential adverse reactions. Additionally, opting for hypoallergenic ingredients, avoiding common irritants, and starting with gentle formulations can help minimize the risk of allergic reactions.

How long can DIY skincare products be stored?

The shelf life of DIY skincare products varies depending on the ingredients used and the presence of preservatives. Natural products without preservatives typically have shorter shelf lives and should be used within a few weeks. Proper storage in airtight containers, away from direct sunlight and heat, can help extend their shelf life.

Can I substitute ingredients in DIY skincare recipes?

Substituting ingredients in DIY skincare recipes is possible, but it may affect the effectiveness and stability of the product. It is important to understand the properties of the original ingredient and its potential alternatives before making substitutions. Modifying recipes should be done cautiously, and adjustments should be made based on research and experimentation.

Can I use DIY skincare alongside commercial products?

Using DIY skincare alongside commercial products is a personal choice. It is important to consider compatibility, potential interactions, and the specific needs of your skin. Some individuals choose to incorporate DIY products as an addition to their existing skincare routine, while others prefer to use them exclusively.

When should I consult a dermatologist or skincare professional?

Consulting a dermatologist or skincare professional is advisable when dealing with severe or persistent skin conditions, allergies, or concerns. They can provide personalized advice, diagnose specific conditions, and guide you in creating an effective skincare routine.

Addressing frequently asked questions in DIY skincare is essential for promoting safe and effective practices. By providing detailed answers to common questions, individuals can make informed decisions, navigate the world of DIY skincare with confidence, and achieve healthier, more radiant skin naturally. It is always important to conduct thorough research, practice good hygiene, and listen to your skin's unique needs throughout your DIY skincare journey.

CHAPTER 8: SUSTAINABILITY AND ECO-FRIENDLY PRACTICES

Importance of sustainable skincare choices

In recent years, there has been a growing awareness of the environmental impact of the beauty industry, prompting individuals to seek sustainable skincare choices. Sustainable skincare refers to the use of products and practices that minimize harm to the environment, promote ethical sourcing, and prioritize long-term ecological balance. Making sustainable skincare choices is not only beneficial for the planet but also for our own well-being. Let's explore the importance of sustainable skincare choices in more detail.

Environmental Impact: The conventional beauty industry often relies on unsustainable practices, including excessive packaging, resource-intensive manufacturing processes, and the use of harmful chemicals. By opting for sustainable skincare choices, such as eco-friendly packaging, biodegradable ingredients, and natural formulations, we can significantly reduce our environmental footprint and contribute to the conservation of natural resources.

Preservation of Biodiversity: Sustainable skincare promotes the use of responsibly sourced ingredients that respect biodiversity and ecosystem health. By supporting brands that prioritize ethical sourcing and fair trade practices, we contribute to the preservation of plant diversity and the protection of indigenous communities that rely on these resources.

Reduction of Waste: The beauty industry generates an enormous amount of waste, from packaging materials to single-use products. Sustainable skincare choices encourage the use of recyclable, reusable, or compostable packaging to minimize waste. Additionally, embracing DIY skincare and minimalism can help reduce the accumulation of unnecessary products and packaging.

Health and Well-being: Conventional skincare products often contain synthetic chemicals that can have long-term detrimental effects on our health and the environment. Sustainable skincare choices prioritize natural and organic ingredients, avoiding harmful substances such as parabens, phthalates, and sulfates. This promotes healthier skin and reduces the risk of allergic reactions or irritations.

Ethical Considerations: Sustainable skincare choices go beyond environmental impact and encompass ethical considerations. By supporting brands that engage in fair trade, use cruelty-free practices, and prioritize transparency in their supply chains, we contribute to a more ethical and responsible industry. This fosters a positive impact on workers' rights, animal welfare, and social justice.

Education and Consumer Awareness: Making sustainable skincare choices encourages a deeper understanding of the products we use and their impact on the planet. It prompts us to become more conscious consumers, seeking information about ingredients, production processes, and the values of the brands we support. This education empowers us to make informed decisions and advocate for change within the beauty industry.

Setting a Positive Example: By making sustainable skincare choices, we inspire others to do the same. Sharing our knowledge, experiences, and recommendations can create a ripple effect, encouraging friends, family, and communities to make more conscious choices in their skincare routines. Collectively, we can drive industry-wide change and encourage brands to adopt more sustainable practices.

The importance of sustainable skincare choices cannot be overstated. By opting for eco-friendly packaging, ethically sourced ingredients, and natural formulations, we can minimize our environmental impact, promote biodiversity, reduce waste, and prioritize our own health and well-being. Making sustainable skincare choices is not just a personal decision but a collective responsibility to protect our planet and build a more sustainable future. Together, we can create a beauty industry that harmonizes with nature and respects the delicate balance of our ecosystems.

Tips for reducing waste and packaging

In our increasingly environmentally conscious world, finding ways to reduce waste and packaging has become a top priority for many individuals. The beauty and skincare industry, in particular, can be a significant contributor to waste generation due to excessive packaging and single-use products. By adopting mindful and sustainable practices, we can make a positive impact and minimize our environmental footprint. Let's explore some tips for reducing waste and packaging in the realm of beauty and skincare.

Choose Minimal Packaging: When selecting skincare products, opt for those with minimal packaging or those packaged in recyclable or biodegradable materials. Look for brands that prioritize eco-friendly packaging options, such as glass, aluminum, or cardboard, which can be easily recycled or repurposed.

Refillable and Reusable Options: Seek out refillable or reusable packaging alternatives. Some companies offer refillable options for skincare products like moisturizers, serums, and even makeup. These containers can be refilled with product from larger, bulk-sized containers, reducing the need for additional packaging.

DIY and Zero-Waste Alternatives: Consider DIY skincare as an alternative to store-bought products. DIY recipes allow you to create personalized skincare solutions using ingredients with minimal packaging or those that can be bought in bulk. Additionally, explore zero-waste options like solid bar cleansers or shampoo bars that eliminate the need for plastic bottles.

Buy in Bulk: Whenever possible, purchase skincare products in bulk sizes. This reduces the amount of packaging per unit of product and can save money in the long run. Remember to transfer the product to smaller, reusable containers for everyday use to avoid waste.

Avoid Single-Use Products: Single-use products, such as face wipes and sheet masks, contribute significantly to waste. Instead, opt for reusable alternatives like muslin cloths, reusable makeup remover pads, or DIY cloth masks. These options can be washed and reused, reducing the amount of waste generated.

Recycle Properly: Familiarize yourself with local recycling guidelines and ensure proper separation and disposal of recyclable packaging materials. Rinse out containers thoroughly and remove any non-recyclable components before recycling. Take the time to educate yourself on what can and cannot be recycled in your area.

Repurpose and Upcycle: Get creative with packaging materials by repurposing them for other uses. Glass jars can be used to store homemade products or for organizing small items. Empty product containers can be repurposed as travel-sized containers or as part of a DIY storage system.

Support Eco-Conscious Brands: Choose to support brands that prioritize sustainable practices and have a commitment to reducing waste and packaging. Look for certifications such as "Cruelty-Free," "Vegan," or "Recyclable Packaging" to ensure your purchasing decisions align with your values.

Spread the Word: Share your knowledge and experiences with others to raise awareness about the importance of reducing waste and packaging in the beauty and skincare industry. Encourage friends, family, and online communities to adopt more sustainable practices and make informed choices.

Continual Learning: Stay informed about new developments in sustainable packaging and waste reduction. Keep up with industry trends and innovations to discover new ways to minimize waste and contribute to a more sustainable future.

Reducing waste and packaging in the beauty and skincare industry requires a conscious effort and a commitment to sustainable practices. By choosing minimal packaging, embracing DIY alternatives, buying in bulk, avoiding single-use products, recycling properly, repurposing packaging materials, and supporting eco-conscious brands, we can make a significant impact on waste reduction. Together, let's take steps towards a more sustainable and mindful approach to beauty and skincare that respects our planet and future generations.

Exploring eco-friendly alternatives

In today's world, there is a growing awareness and concern for the environment, leading more individuals to seek eco-friendly alternatives in various aspects of their lives. Exploring eco-friendly alternatives involves making conscious choices that prioritize sustainability, reduce waste, and minimize the ecological impact of our actions. When it comes to everyday practices, including skincare, there are several ways to embrace eco-friendly alternatives.

One key aspect of exploring eco-friendly alternatives is considering the materials used in the products we use. Instead of opting for conventional materials that have a detrimental impact on the environment, we can choose products made from sustainable materials. For example, bamboo is a fast-growing and renewable resource that can be used in packaging or as a material for skincare tools like brushes or washcloths. Organic cotton is another sustainable option, as it is grown without the use of harmful pesticides.

Another important aspect of eco-friendly alternatives is reducing waste, particularly in packaging. Many conventional skincare products come in excessive packaging that ends up in landfills or contributes to pollution. By seeking out products with minimal or plastic-free packaging, we can reduce our environmental footprint. Brands that prioritize sustainable packaging options, such as glass jars or paperboard tubes, offer viable alternatives to plastic containers.

In addition to reducing waste, embracing reusable options is a significant step towards eco-friendliness. Instead of using single-use items like cotton pads or makeup wipes, reusable alternatives like cotton or bamboo pads can be washed and reused multiple times, reducing waste generation. Similarly, investing in refillable containers for skincare products allows us to reduce the consumption of single-use plastic bottles.

Exploring eco-friendly alternatives also involves considering the ingredients used in skincare products. Opting for natural, organic, and biodegradable ingredients helps minimize the release of harmful chemicals into the environment. Additionally, choosing products from ethical and cruelty-free brands ensures that no animal testing or exploitation is involved.

Water conservation is another aspect of eco-friendly alternatives. By reducing water usage in our skincare routine, such as taking shorter showers or turning off the tap while cleansing or applying products, we can conserve this precious resource. Waterless skincare options, which do not require rinsing, are also gaining popularity as sustainable alternatives.

Engaging in community initiatives and supporting local sustainable businesses further promotes eco-friendly alternatives. Participating in recycling programs, shopping at farmers' markets or local artisans who use sustainable practices, and sharing knowledge about eco-friendly alternatives with friends and family contribute to creating a more sustainable community.

Education and awareness play a vital role in exploring eco-friendly alternatives. Staying informed about sustainable practices, reading about environmental issues, and engaging in discussions help us make informed choices and inspire others to do the same. Sharing information through social media, attending sustainability events, or joining online communities focused on eco-friendly living can amplify our impact.

Exploring eco-friendly alternatives in skincare and everyday practices is crucial for reducing our environmental footprint and preserving the planet. By considering sustainable materials, reducing waste, embracing reusability, choosing natural ingredients, conserving water, supporting local initiatives, and staying educated, we can make a positive impact on the environment and inspire others to do the same. Together, we can create a more sustainable future for generations to come.

CHAPTER 9: SAFETY CONSIDERATIONS AND ALLERGIES

Identifying potential allergies and sensitivities

Allergies and sensitivities to certain substances can have a significant impact on our overall health and well-being. In the context of skincare, it is crucial to identify potential allergies and sensitivities to specific ingredients to ensure the safety and effectiveness of the products we use. Here is a detailed explanation of how to identify potential allergies and sensitivities:

Understanding Allergies and Sensitivities: Allergies and sensitivities are immune system reactions, but they differ in intensity and mechanism. Allergies involve a hypersensitive immune response to an allergen, leading to immediate symptoms like itching, redness, or swelling. Sensitivities, on the other hand, are non-immune reactions that can manifest as delayed or chronic symptoms like skin irritation, dryness, or rash.

Patch Testing: Patch testing is a common method used to identify allergies and sensitivities. It involves applying small amounts of the product or ingredient to a patch of skin, usually on the inner forearm or behind the ear, and monitoring the area for any adverse reactions. Patch testing is particularly important when using new products or ingredients to determine if they cause any allergic or sensitive reactions.

Observing Immediate Reactions: Pay close attention to your skin's immediate reaction after applying a new product. Look for signs of redness, itching, swelling, or a burning sensation. These immediate reactions may indicate an allergic response. If you experience such symptoms, discontinue use of the product and consult a healthcare professional for further evaluation.

Monitoring Delayed Reactions: Some allergic or sensitive reactions may not appear immediately but can develop over time with repeated exposure to an allergen or irritant. Keep track of any delayed skin reactions, such as persistent dryness, flakiness, or rashes that appear hours or even days after using a particular product. These delayed reactions may indicate a sensitivity, and it is advisable to discontinue use and seek professional advice.

Keeping a Skincare Diary: Maintaining a skincare diary can be helpful in identifying potential allergies and sensitivities. Record the products you use, along with any symptoms or reactions you experience. This record can provide valuable insights, especially when trying to pinpoint the specific ingredient or product causing the reaction. Share this information with a dermatologist or allergist for a thorough evaluation.

Professional Consultation: If you suspect allergies or sensitivities, it is advisable to consult a dermatologist or allergist for an accurate diagnosis. They can perform specific tests, such as patch testing or blood tests, to identify allergens or sensitizing substances. These professionals can provide guidance on managing your skincare routine and recommend alternative products or ingredients that are safe for your specific needs.

Reading Ingredient Labels: Familiarize yourself with common allergens or irritants found in skincare products. Look for ingredient labels that provide transparency about the product's composition. Be cautious if you have known allergies to substances like fragrances, preservatives (e.g., parabens), certain botanical extracts, or specific chemicals (e.g., formaldehyde releasers). Avoid products that contain these potential allergens or irritants to minimize the risk of adverse reactions.

Gradual Introduction of New Products: When introducing new skincare products, especially if you have a history of allergies or sensitivities, do so gradually. Start by patch testing and gradually increase usage over a few days, observing for any adverse reactions. This approach allows you to identify and address any potential sensitivities before fully incorporating the product into your routine.

Personalized Approach: Skincare is highly individual, and what works for one person may not work for another. Understanding your skin's unique needs and potential allergies or sensitivities is crucial for creating a personalized skincare routine. This may involve avoiding certain ingredients or using products specifically formulated for sensitive skin. Consulting a skincare professional can help you tailor your routine to your specific concerns and minimize the risk of adverse reactions.

Identifying potential allergies and sensitivities in skincare is essential for maintaining healthy and radiant skin. By understanding the differences between allergies and sensitivities, conducting patch tests, observing immediate and delayed reactions, keeping a skincare diary, seeking professional consultation, reading ingredient labels, gradually introducing new products, and adopting a personalized approach, you can navigate your skincare journey with confidence and minimize the risk of adverse reactions. Prioritizing your skin's health and well-being is

key to achieving a skincare routine that suits your individual needs.

Patch testing and safety precautions

Patch testing is a method used to assess potential allergies or sensitivities to skincare products or ingredients. It involves applying a small amount of the product or ingredient to a specific area of the skin and observing any adverse reactions over a designated period. Patch testing is an essential step in skincare to ensure safety and identify potential irritants or allergens that may cause skin reactions.

When conducting a patch test, it is important to choose a small, unaffected area of skin that is easily accessible and easily observed. Common areas for patch testing include the inner forearm, behind the ear, or the upper back. Avoid areas that are sunburned, irritated, or have cuts or wounds.

Before applying the patch test, cleanse the chosen area with mild soap and water. Ensure the skin is thoroughly dry before proceeding. Then, apply a small amount of the product or ingredient onto the skin, spreading it evenly. Use a sterile cotton swab or a clean fingertip for application.

Once applied, secure the area with a hypoallergenic adhesive patch or medical tape. Leave the patch on for the recommended time, usually 24 to 48 hours, without getting it wet or exposing it to excessive sweating. During this period, it is essential to avoid activities that may cause friction or irritation to the patch test area.

After the designated period, carefully remove the patch and examine the skin for any signs of adverse reactions. Look for redness, itching, swelling, or any other noticeable changes. Document any reactions and note their severity and location.

It is important to interpret the results of the patch test accurately. Positive reactions may indicate an allergy or sensitivity to the tested product or ingredient. In such cases, it is advisable to discontinue using the product or avoid the specific ingredient to prevent further skin reactions.

To ensure safety during patch testing, it is crucial to observe several precautions. First, only patch test one product or ingredient at a time to accurately identify the cause of any reactions. If multiple products are tested simultaneously, it becomes challenging to determine which one is causing the reaction.

Additionally, it is important to follow the instructions regarding the patch test duration and any specific precautions recommended. Adhering to the recommended time frame ensures sufficient exposure for potential reactions to occur.

If you have a history of severe allergies or sensitivities, it is advisable to consult a dermatologist or allergist before conducting patch testing. They can provide guidance and recommend specific protocols based on your individual needs.

Patch testing is an important safety measure in skincare to identify potential allergies or sensitivities. By following proper procedures, selecting an appropriate test area, applying the product or ingredient, securing the patch, observing for reactions, and interpreting the results accurately, you can effectively assess the safety of skincare products and ingredients and make informed decisions about your skincare routine.

When it comes to skincare, consulting professionals can provide valuable guidance and expertise, particularly in complex or severe cases. Here is a detailed explanation of when and why it is important to seek professional advice:

Dermatologists: Dermatologists are medical doctors who specialize in diagnosing and treating skin conditions. If you have persistent or severe skin issues that are not improving with over-the-counter remedies, it is advisable to consult a dermatologist. They can evaluate your skin, identify underlying causes, and recommend appropriate treatments or prescriptions. Dermatologists can also offer personalized advice tailored to your specific skin concerns, ensuring safe and effective skincare practices.

Allergists: Allergists specialize in identifying and managing allergic reactions. If you suspect that your skin issues are due to allergies or sensitivities, an allergist can help pinpoint the specific allergens causing the reactions. They can conduct tests, such as patch testing or blood tests, to determine the substances triggering your skin symptoms. With this information, they can provide targeted recommendations to help you avoid allergens and manage your skincare routine effectively.

Estheticians: Estheticians are skincare professionals trained in various aspects of skincare, including analyzing skin conditions and providing customized treatments. They can assess your skin's needs, recommend appropriate products, and perform treatments such as facials or peels. Estheticians can also provide advice on skincare routines, including cleansing, exfoliation, and moisturizing. While estheticians cannot diagnose or treat medical conditions, they can play a valuable role in improving your skin's health and appearance.

Cosmetic Scientists: Cosmetic scientists specialize in formulating skincare products and understanding the interactions between ingredients and the skin. They possess in-depth knowledge of skincare ingredients, their efficacy, and potential side effects. Consulting a cosmetic scientist can be beneficial if you have specific concerns about ingredient interactions, formulation techniques, or the safety of DIY skincare recipes. They can provide expert advice on modifying or developing skincare formulations to suit your needs.

Pharmacists: Pharmacists are healthcare professionals who are well-versed in medications and their potential effects on the body. If you are using prescription medications for skin conditions or incorporating skincare products alongside other medications, consulting a pharmacist is important. They can advise on possible drug interactions or contraindications, ensuring the compatibility and safety of your skincare routine with your medications.

Mental Health Professionals: Sometimes, skincare concerns can have an emotional impact, leading to feelings of low self-esteem or body image issues. In such cases, seeking support from mental health professionals, such as therapists or counselors, can be helpful. They can address the emotional aspects of skincare struggles and provide coping strategies to improve overall well-being.

When consulting professionals, it is important to provide them with a comprehensive medical history, including any existing conditions, allergies, or medications you are taking. This information helps them make accurate assessments and provide tailored advice.

Consulting professionals when needed can greatly benefit your skincare journey. Dermatologists, allergists, estheticians, cosmetic scientists, pharmacists, and mental health professionals can offer specialized expertise, diagnose underlying issues, recommend appropriate treatments, provide personalized skincare advice, and ensure the safety and efficacy of your skincare routine. By seeking professional guidance, you can address complex skin concerns, make informed decisions, and achieve optimal skin health.

CHAPTER 10: INCORPORATING SKINCARE INTO A HEALTHY LIFESTYLE

Importance of a holistic approach to skin-care

A holistic approach to skincare recognizes that the health and appearance of our skin are influenced by various interconnected factors. It goes beyond surface-level treatments and addresses the underlying causes of skin issues, emphasizing overall well-being and balance. Here is a detailed explanation of why adopting a holistic approach to skincare is crucial:

Mind-Body Connection: Our mental and emotional well-being directly impacts our skin health. Stress, anxiety, and other psychological factors can trigger skin conditions like acne, eczema, or psoriasis. By addressing stress management techniques, practicing mindfulness, and seeking emotional support, we can improve our skin's overall health.

Nutrition and Hydration: What we consume affects the condition of our skin. A holistic approach encourages a nutrient-rich diet that includes fruits, vegetables, whole grains, lean proteins, and healthy fats. Proper hydration is also essential to maintain skin hydration and overall skin health. By nourishing our bodies from within, we promote healthy skin from the inside out.

Lifestyle Factors: Sleep, exercise, and habits such as smoking or excessive alcohol consumption can impact skin health. Adequate sleep allows for proper skin repair and rejuvenation, while regular exercise promotes circulation, which benefits the skin. Avoiding harmful habits and adopting a healthy lifestyle contribute to overall skin well-being.

Environmental Factors: Environmental elements like pollution, sun exposure, and harsh weather conditions can damage the skin. A holistic approach encourages protective measures, such as wearing sunscreen, using natural and eco-friendly skincare products, and practicing good environmental habits to minimize exposure to harmful substances.

Skincare Routine: A holistic skincare routine focuses on using products and ingredients that are gentle, natural, and free from harsh chemicals. It emphasizes the importance of understanding our skin's specific needs and selecting products accordingly. A holistic approach encourages regular cleansing, exfoliating, moisturizing, and sun protection as part of a comprehensive skincare regimen.

Emotional Well-being: Skin concerns can impact self-esteem and body image. A holistic approach recognizes the emotional aspect of skincare and encourages self-acceptance and self-care practices. By nurturing a positive self-image and practicing self-love, we enhance our overall well-being and promote healthy skin.

Regular Check-ups: Regular visits to dermatologists or skincare professionals are essential to monitor skin health, address concerns, and receive professional advice. They can provide insights into specific skin conditions, recommend appropriate treatments, and ensure early detection of any potential issues.

By adopting a holistic approach to skincare, we acknowledge the interconnectedness of our physical, mental, and emotional well-being. It allows us to address the root causes of skin concerns, promote overall health, and achieve radiant, healthy skin. Taking care of our skin from a holistic perspective not only enhances its appearance but also contributes to our overall wellness and quality of life.

Achieving healthy and radiant skin goes beyond the use of skincare products alone. It involves creating a holistic approach that combines skincare, nutrition, and exercise. By understanding the interconnectedness of these factors, you can promote optimal skin health and overall well-being.

Nutrition plays a vital role in supporting skin health. A well-balanced diet rich in fruits, vegetables, whole grains, lean proteins, and healthy fats provides essential vitamins, minerals, antioxidants, and nutrients that nourish the skin from within. Specific nutrients like vitamins A, C, and E, zinc, and omega-3 fatty acids are known to support skin health, collagen production, and protection against environmental damage. Incorporating these nutrient-dense foods into your daily meals can promote a healthy complexion and combat skin issues.

Hydration is crucial for maintaining healthy skin. Drinking an adequate amount of water throughout the day helps to keep your skin hydrated, plump, and radiant. Additionally, certain foods, such as cucumbers, watermelon, and citrus fruits, have high water content and can contribute to your overall hydration.

Exercise plays a significant role in promoting skin health. Regular physical activity improves blood circulation, delivering oxygen and nutrients to the skin while removing toxins and waste products. This increased blood flow helps nourish the skin cells, promotes a healthy complexion, and enhances the skin's natural detoxification process. Engaging in activities like jogging, swimming, yoga, or strength training can contribute to healthier and more vibrant skin.

Stress reduction is also essential for maintaining skin health. Exercise serves as an effective stress reliever, releasing endorphins and reducing stress levels. High-stress levels can lead to inflammation, hormonal imbalances, and skin conditions like acne or eczema. By incorporating exercise into your routine, you can manage stress levels, promote relaxation, and support a healthier complexion.

Taking a personalized approach is key when balancing skincare with nutrition and exercise. Each person's skin is unique, and what works for one individual may not work for another. It's important to listen to your body, pay attention to how certain foods and activities affect your skin, and make adjustments accordingly. Consulting with healthcare professionals, such as dermatologists or nutritionists, can provide valuable insights and guidance tailored to your specific needs.

Balancing skincare with nutrition and exercise is a holistic approach that addresses skin health from multiple angles. By nourishing your body with a nutrient-rich diet, staying hydrated, engaging in regular physical activity, and managing stress levels, you create a strong foundation for healthy, glowing skin. Remember to embrace a personalized approach and make choices that support your individual skin needs.

Self-care practices for overall well-being

Self-care practices are vital for promoting overall well-being and maintaining a healthy and balanced life. Taking care of yourself goes beyond physical health; it encompasses nurturing your mental, emotional, and spiritual well-being. One essential self-care practice is setting aside time for relaxation and rejuvenation. This could involve activities such as reading a book, taking a walk in nature, or engaging in a hobby that brings you joy.

Prioritizing self-care also means learning to establish boundaries and saying no when necessary. It's important to recognize your limits and avoid overcommitting yourself, as this can lead to stress and burnout. By setting boundaries, you create space for self-care and protect your mental and emotional energy.

Taking care of your physical health is another crucial aspect of self-care. This includes regular exercise to keep your body strong and energized. Find physical activities that you enjoy, whether it's dancing, yoga, or going for a run. Additionally, nourishing your body with nutritious foods and staying hydrated supports overall well-being.

Emotional well-being is also a key component of self-care. This involves practicing self-compassion, being kind to yourself, and managing stress effectively. Engaging in activities that help you process and express your emotions, such as journaling or talking to a trusted friend or therapist, can be beneficial.

Self-care extends beyond individual practices; it also involves cultivating meaningful connections and nurturing relationships. Spending quality time with loved ones, engaging in activities that promote social connection, and seeking support when needed are essential for emotional well-being.

Lastly, self-care is about listening to your intuition and honoring your needs. Pay attention to your inner voice and give yourself permission to prioritize self-care without guilt. Remember, self-care is not selfish but necessary for maintaining overall well-being and showing up as your best self in all areas of life.

CONCLUSION

Recap of key points and takeaways

In summary, DIY skincare offers a wonderful opportunity to take control of your skincare routine and customize products using natural ingredients. Here are the key points and takeaways to remember:

Firstly, DIY skincare allows you to avoid potentially harmful ingredients commonly found in commercial products. By using natural ingredients, you can minimize the exposure to harsh chemicals and irritants, promoting healthier skin.

Secondly, DIY skincare provides the flexibility to tailor products to your specific needs. Whether you have dry skin, oily skin, acne-prone skin, or aging skin, you can modify recipes and ingredients to address your unique concerns and achieve the desired results.

It's important to note that understanding your skin type and specific needs is crucial when selecting and modifying DIY skincare recipes. Take the time to learn about your skin's characteristics, such as oiliness, sensitivity, or hydration levels, so you can make informed decisions about the ingredients and formulations that will work best for you.

Experimentation is key when creating DIY skincare products. Don't be afraid to try different ingredients and combinations to find what works best for your skin. Keep in mind that everyone's skin is unique, so what works for others may not necessarily work for you.

Additionally, maintaining proper hygiene and safety measures is essential in DIY skincare. Make sure to store your homemade products properly, follow good manufacturing practices, and conduct patch tests to check for any adverse reactions before using a new product on your entire face or body.

Lastly, remember that DIY skincare is not a substitute for professional advice. If you have severe skin conditions or concerns, it's always wise to consult a dermatologist or skincare professional who can provide personalized guidance and recommendations.

In conclusion, DIY skincare can be a rewarding and empowering journey, allowing you to take charge of your skincare routine and use natural ingredients that suit your skin's unique needs. By understanding your skin, experimenting with ingredients, and maintaining proper hygiene and safety, you can create effective and personalized skincare products. However, it's important to stay informed, seek professional guidance when needed, and remember that self-care is a holistic approach that encompasses more than just skincare – it also involves overall well-being and self-nurturing.

Encouragement to start the journey of DIY natural skincare

Embarking on the journey of DIY natural skincare is an exciting and empowering endeavor. It offers the opportunity to take control of what you put on your skin, customize products to your specific needs, and indulge in the beauty and benefits of natural ingredients. If you're considering starting this journey, here's some encouragement to help you take that first step.

DIY natural skincare allows you to develop a deeper connection with your skin. By becoming more involved in the creation of your skincare products, you gain a better understanding of your skin's unique needs and can tailor your routine accordingly. It's a chance to truly listen to your skin and respond with ingredients that nourish and support its health.

DIY natural skincare is a creative outlet that allows you to experiment with various ingredients and formulations. You can explore the vast world of botanicals, oils, herbs, and essential oils, discovering the amazing benefits they can offer to your skin. It's an opportunity to tap into your creativity and develop personalized products that cater to your preferences and desired results.

DIY natural skincare also encourages sustainability and conscious consumption. By making your own products, you have the power to reduce packaging waste, minimize your environmental footprint, and support a more eco-friendly approach to skincare. You can choose organic, ethically sourced ingredients and minimize your reliance on single-use plastic containers.

Embracing DIY natural skincare fosters a sense of empowerment and self-care. It's an act of self-love and self-care to devote time and attention to nurturing your skin with wholesome, natural ingredients. It can become a mindful and soothing ritual that promotes overall well-being, allowing you to reconnect with yourself and indulge in moments of relaxation and self-nurturing.

So, if you're ready to embark on this journey, gather your ingredients, educate yourself about different ingredients and their benefits, and start experimenting. Remember, it's a journey of self-discovery and continuous learning. Be patient, embrace the process, and enjoy the satisfaction of creating skincare products that are uniquely yours.

By embracing DIY natural skincare, you are taking a step towards a healthier, more sustainable, and more conscious approach to caring for your skin. Your skin will thank you for the nourishment and love you provide, and you'll find joy and fulfillment in the journey of crafting your own personalized skincare routine.

Final thoughts and resources for further exploration

In conclusion, venturing into the world of DIY natural skincare is a wonderful way to connect with your skin, embrace sustainable practices, and create products that cater to your unique needs. As you embark on this journey, remember to prioritize safety, conduct patch tests, and consult professionals when needed. The key is to be open to experimentation and to listen to your skin's feedback along the way.

To further your exploration and knowledge, there are various resources available. Online communities, forums, and social media platforms dedicated to natural skincare offer a wealth of information, tips, and insights from fellow DIY enthusiasts. Books, blogs, and websites authored by skincare experts and holistic practitioners can also provide valuable guidance and inspiration.

Additionally, consider attending workshops or classes on natural skincare formulation. These hands-on experiences can deepen your understanding of ingredients, techniques, and safety precautions, while also providing an opportunity to connect with like-minded individuals.

When sourcing ingredients, opt for reputable suppliers that offer organic, sustainably sourced, and cruelty-free options. Look for certifications such as USDA organic or Fair Trade to ensure the quality and ethical sourcing of your ingredients.

Remember, the journey of DIY natural skincare is a continuous learning process. Be open to adapting your recipes and routines as you discover what works best for your skin. Pay attention to the needs and changes of your skin over time, as it may require adjustments to the products you create.

Above all, enjoy the process and embrace the self-care aspect of DIY natural skincare. Take pleasure in creating products that are not only beneficial for your skin but also provide moments of relaxation, indulgence and self-nurturing.

As you venture forth on this journey, may your exploration of DIY natural skincare bring you joy, radiant skin and a deeper connection with the beauty and wisdom of nature.

ABOUT THE AUTHOR

Elara Finch is a passionate skincare enthusiast, writer, and advocate for natural and sustainable beauty practices. With a deep fascination for the science behind skincare and a commitment to promoting healthy and mindful living, Elara Finch has dedicated years to researching and exploring the world of natural skincare.

Inspired by a personal journey of discovering the transformative power of DIY skincare, Elara Finch has become a trusted resource for those seeking to enhance their skincare routines using homemade products. Through extensive experimentation and a thorough understanding of ingredients, Elara Finch has developed a wealth of knowledge in formulating effective and nourishing skincare solutions.

Beyond writing, Elara Finch actively engages in the skincare community, participating in workshops, conferences, and ongoing education to stay updated on the latest trends and advancements in natural skincare. Through her work, Elara Finch aims to empower individuals to take control of their skincare journey, embracing the power of natural ingredients and the joy of creating personalized products.

When not immersed in the world of skincare, Elara Finch enjoys spending time outdoors, practicing yoga, and experimenting with new recipes in the kitchen. She believe that true beauty begins from within and that caring for oneself holistically is the key to achieving radiant and healthy skin.